Clinical Practice in Urology
Series Editor: Geoffrey D. Chisholm

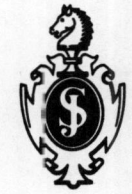

Clinical Practice in Urology
Series Editor: Geoffrey D. Chisholm

Practical Urology in Spinal Cord Injury

Edited by

Keith F. Parsons and John M. Fitzpatrick

With 14 Figures

Springer-Verlag London Ltd.

Keith F. Parsons, MB, ChB, FRCSE, FRCS
Consultant Urological Surgeon,
Royal Liverpool Hospital University NHS Trust, Prescott Street,
Liverpool L7 8XP, UK

John M. Fitzpatrick, MCh, FRCSI
Professor of Surgery and Consultant Urological Surgeon,
Mater Misericordiae Hospital and University College, 47 Eccles
Street, Dublin, Ireland

Series Editor
Geoffrey D. Chisholm, ChM, FRCS, FRCSEd
Professor of Surgery, University of Edinburgh
and Consultant Urological Surgeon, Western General Hospital,
Edinburgh, Scotland

ISBN 978-1-4471-1862-6   ISBN 978-1-4471-1860-2 (eBook)
DOI 10.1007/978-1-4471-1860-2

ISBN 3-540-19676-5 Springer-Verlag Berlin Heidelberg New York
ISBN 0-387-19676-5 Springer-Verlag New York Berlin Heidelberg

British Library Cataloguing in Publication Data
Practical urology in spinal cord injury.
1. Humans. Urinary Tract. Diagnosis
I. Parsons, Keith F.   II Fitzpatrick, John M.   III. Series
616.6
ISBN 0-540-19676-5

Library of Congress Cataloguing-in-Publication Data
Practical urology in spinal cord injury/edited by Keith F. Parsons and John M.
Fitzpatrick.
p.   cm. – (Clinical practice in urology)
Includes index.
ISBN 0-540-19676-5 (alk. paper). – ISBN 0-387-19676-5 (alk. paper)
1. Spinal cord—Wounds and injuries—Complications and sequelae.
2. Urinary organs—Diseases.   I. Parsons, Keith F., 1947–.   II Fitzpatrick, John M.
III. Series
[DNLM: 1. Spinal Cord Injuries--complications.   2. Urologic Diseases--
therapy.   WJ 166 P895]
RD594.3.P73 1991
617.4'82044--dc20
DNLM/DLC
for Library of Congress   91-4645
                                                                     CIP

Typeset by Electronic Village, Richmond, UK
2128/3830-543210   Printed on acid-free paper

Series Editor's Foreword

In keeping with the aims of other books in this Series the Editors have concentrated on the practical aspects of management – in this case of the urinary tract in patients with spinal cord injury. It is well accepted that the management of such patients is best done by those with special experience in this field. Nevertheless, it is essential that urologists should be well informed on matters relating to the neuropathic urinary tract since not all patients will be managed in special centres and, whether their problems are acute or chronic, the wrong clinical decision can lead them into a lifetime of problems.

The plan of this book is directed towards examining particular problems and providing definitive answers. Even in this enlightened age of medical progress there are many clinical situations where there is often a choice of treatment. Readers of this Series will be aware that, despite an apparent abundance of information on a topic, it is sometimes not possible to reach a firm conclusion on a management problem. Keith Parsons and John Fitzpatrick are to be congratulated on ensuring that for this subject there are good clear guidelines. The data in the book are up to date and the excellent approach to the subject makes it a valuable addition to Clinical Practice in Urology.

Edinburgh   Geoffrey D. Chisholm
February 1991

Preface

There is no doubt that the management of the neuropathic urinary tract is a highly sophisticated specialty and much has been written on the topic over the years. Indeed it is largely because of detailed attention to the urinary tract that the life expectancy of patients with spinal cord injury has been increased and their quality of life improved. Attention largely has been focused quite properly on the disordered function of the bladder and urethra and from this has evolved a much greater understanding of the pathophysiology of micturition. Yet the whole of the urinary tract is potentially affected by vesico-urethral neuropathy and the sequelae of midline neuropathic obstruction on the rest of the urinary tract is well recognised.

From the practical standpoint, clinicians who have to deal on occasions with patients with spinal cord injury who come under their care either in the acute phase or at any stage, may find it difficult to translocate this mountain of knowledge into practical terms to the best advantage of their patient.

Experience has shown that there are several aspects of the neuropathic urinary tract with which these patients present and the editors have therefore asked their contributors to address themselves to these specific circumstances and to give didactic and practical guidelines as to how each should be managed on the basis of their authoritative and renowned expertise in the field.

Thus it is hoped that this volume will serve as a helpful practical guide to clinicians charged with the management of the urinary tract in patients with spinal cord injury.

Liverpool and Dublin 1990   Keith F. Parsons
                                                      John M. Fitzpatrick

Contents

Contributors

E. P. Arnold, MD, FRCS
Associate Professor of Urology, Christchurch Hospital, Canterbury, New Zealand

C. J. Bennett, MD
Assistant Professor, Department of Urology, University of Southern California, Los Angeles, California, USA

J. M. Fitzpatrick, MCh, FRCSI
Professsor of Surgery and Consultant Urologist,
Mater Misericordiae Hospital and University College, Dublin, Ireland

B. P. Gardner, MA, MRCP(UK), FRCS
Consultant Surgeon in Spinal Injuries, National Spinal Injuries Centre, Stoke Mandeville Hospital, Aylesbury,
Buckinghamshire, UK

C. A. Glass, PhD
Clinical Psychologist, Mersey Regional Spinal Injuries Centre, General Infirmary, Southport, Merseyside, UK

R. J. Krane, MD
Professor and Chairman, Department of Urology,
Boston University Medical Center,
Boston, Massachusetts, USA

K. R. Krishnan, MBChB, FRCS
Director, Mersey Regional Spinal Injuries Centre,
General Infirmary, Southport, Merseyside, UK

E. J. McGuire, MD
Professor and Chairman, Department of Urology, University of Michigan Medical Center, Ann Arbor, Michigan, USA

D. A. Ohl, MD
Instructor, Section of Urology, Department of Surgery, University
of Michigan Medical Center, Ann Arbor, Michigan, USA

K. F. Parsons, MBChB, FRCSE, FRCS
Consultant Urological Surgeon, Royal Liverpool University
Hospital NHS Trust and Mersey Regional Spinal Injuries Centre,
General Infirmary, Southport, and Director of Urological Studies,
University of Liverpool, UK

P. C. Ryan MB, FRCSI
Senior Registrar in Urology, Mater Misericordiae Hospital, Dublin,
Ireland

D. R. Staskin, MD
Assistant Professor of Urology, Beth Israel Hospital, Harvard
Medical School, Boston, Massachusetts, USA

J.W.H. Watt, MD, FFARCS
Consultant Anaesthetist, Mersey Regional Spinal Injuries Centre,
General Infirmary, Southport, Merseyside, UK

Chapter 1

General Considerations in the Management of the Urinary Tract

K.R. Krishnan

High spinal cord injury is the most formidable of all non-fatal injuries producing profound physical disability and radical change in the pattern of life of the sufferer. The dysfunction is not just confined to motor power. The totality of physiological disadvantages consist of sensory deprivation, abolition of bladder and bowel control and sexual function, autonomic decentralisation with deranged thermoregulation and a fragile homeostasis. Almost invariably there is no major mental or emotional deficit due to brain injury and it is this that makes spinal injury a particularly distressing experience. Lack of cosmetic disadvantage, an essentially non-progressive neurological dysfunction and, during the past three or four decades, an exceptionally good life expectancy, have made people with spinal cord injury more in control of their lives than most others with serious physical disability. Such control of life, not unnaturally, increases expectation and discernment of the medical treatment that is offered. It is of concern that this challenge is not always effectively met by the medical profession due to lack of insight into the complex physiological changes produced by spinal cord transection and its social and economic implications.

Though spinal cord injury had been well documented in medical history and the appalling tragedy of the fate of the spinally injured during the 1914–1918 war had caused great concern, it was only during the second world war beginning in 1939 that specialised centres for treatment were established. Without such centres the phenomenal reduction in morbidity with restoration of quality of life and much improved life expectancy after spinal cord injury would not have been possible.

The vast majority of patients are aware of the broad implications and serious degree of disability that are characteristic of spinal injury. In a recent survey of patients in the Southport centre, 95% had much understanding of the probable implications of their injury within the first two days and most whilst they were still at the site of the accident. Perception of the nature of disability is of crucial significance to the injured person in the acute phase and during the challenging time of rehabilitation when a new role in life has to be established. The mental response to sudden profound physical disability is dominated and determined by:

1. Sensory deprivation producing total inability to perceive what is being done to one's body and disorientation, both spatial and temporal.
2. An exaggerated fear and preoccupation with the probability of lack of control of urinary bladder and bowels and, by inference, of sexual paralysis and impotence in the male.
3. A global psychological effect of being severely disabled and not in control of one's life.

The intensity of this emotional response and expectation is not often perceived by staff in a general traumatology unit.

In a complete spinal cord injury the "spinal shock" is characterised by global atonia, anaesthesia and areflexia below the level of the lesion. This is manifest in the urinary tract by paralysis of the detrusor muscle and consequent adynamic urinary retention. There are occasions when urinary retention may be the most significant or indeed the only abnormality that suggests a spinal cord injury. Important among such clinical states are:

1. Brain injury or alcohol intoxication producing lowered level of consciousness. An unconscious patient lying in a dry bed for several hours must arouse the probability of spinal cord injury. There may be priapism due to abolition of tone of smooth muscles and passive engorgement of corpora cavernosa.
2. In elderly persons with degenerative disease of the vertebral column or advanced ankylosing spondylitis there is a substantial predisposition for spinal cord injury. There may be a very delicate balance between detrusor power and bladder outlet resistance and even a very incomplete spinal injury may precipitate decompensation and urinary retention.
3. In multiple injuries with fractures of the pelvis or of lower limb long bones, particularly if associated with brain injury, routine catheterisation may be done as part of immediate orthopaedic treatment and the diagnosis of spinal cord injury and neuropathic bladder may be missed during this crucial period.

Accurate and comprehensive neurological assessment in the accident department is therefore fundamental to early diagnosis of bladder dysfunction in spinal injury. The presence of the bulbo-cavernosus reflex denoting continuing function of lower sacral segments is of vital significance in planning treatment and giving a prognosis. This reflex is elicited by a brisk pinching of the glans penis which provokes a contraction of the peri-anal muscles which can readily be seen. In females the same reflex can be observed by pinching the clitoris or, rather more easily, by a single gentle tug on a balloon catheter. The afferent and efferent limbs are in the pudendal nerves and integrity of the conus medullaris, particularly the S2–S4 spinal segments, is required for the reflex to be seen. If present, it can be inferred that the conus parasympathetic micturition centre is intact. Even in unconscious patients a diagnosis of spinal cord damage ought to be possible if there is adequate awareness and accurate neurological examination.

Substantial disruption of the architecture of the vertebral column may exist without overt spinal cord damage. Such disruption in the lower cervical vertebral column is often missed due to inadequate radiography. It is mandatory to visualise the cervico-dorsal junction in all cases of suspected spinal cord injury.

The duration of spinal shock much depends on effective correction of physiological alteration and prompt and appropriate treatment to prevent complications. Allowing the neuropathic bladder to remain severely distended for more than two or three hours may delay return of reflex activity and prolong the time when invasive procedures are necessary to keep the bladder deflated, thereby increasing risk of urinary tract infection. Unfortunately over-distension of the urinary bladder is allowed to occur far too often. A system of management of residual neurological dysfunction as it affects the urinary tract will depend much on the standard of urological care during the acute and early stages. Technological advances in materials and manufacture of catheters, availability of sophisticated urodynamic studies and better understanding of the pathophysiology of the neuropathic urinary tract have enabled the planning of treatment with logic and precision at this critical stage.

Educating disabled persons, their families, nurses and physicians in the community about the vagaries of the neuropathic urinary tract must be an integral part of a rehabilitation programme specifically designed for an individual. Such a programme must be realistic and relevant to the social, economic and cultural implications of an individual's disability. The aim of rehabilitation is to minimise the disabled person's dependence on others and to attain control of life as much and as soon as possible. A fully rehabilitated person is therefore very conversant with the ergonomics specific to him and is inclined to control his environment to compensate for his vulnerability. Such a situation often produces conflict in an establishment where dependence on staff, particularly nurses, is the working pattern which is encouraged and any change in the established system is frowned upon.

Management of the neuropathic urinary tract requires expertise unfamiliar to a "general" urologist in isolation. Only a dedicated urologist who is part of a therapeutic team in a specialised centre that can offer comprehensive advice and support will be able to provide the necessary skill and insight in determining treatment in the acute phase and during rehabilitation. It is difficult to be dogmatic about the frequency and nature of review after discharge from hospital and much will depend on what state a particular urinary tract has been stabilised. Regular annual imaging by ultrasound, radioisotope scans or conventional contrast studies is essential particularly if there is evidence of recurrent urinary tract infection. Substantial structural changes in the urinary tract with or without uretero-vesical incompetence can occur in a relatively short time. Anyone with manifest structural changes should be strictly monitored, the frequency determined by the extent and rapidity of progression and clinical history. Whatever the system is, close co-ordination between the disabled person, the family medical practitioner, community nurses and the spinal injuries centre is the most important single factor in the discipline of continued care.

It is as vital to have microbiological tests and prompt and effective treatment with appropriate chemotherapeutic agents or antibiotics, as indeed it is to discourage therapy by powerful antibiotics without accurate screening. There must be a strict protocol for collection of urine specimens and insight into the part played by urethral contaminants. In a person with abolition of pain sensitivity and altered thermoregulation there may be delay in recognising insidious septicaemia. Seeking prompt advice should be actively encouraged and there should be no hesitation to re-admit to hospital.

Endourological and percutaneous procedures and lithotripsy have made the treatment of complications less time consuming and less morbid and the logistics of offering prompt, radical and effective measures to a large patient population, more manageable. Such treatments, however, should only be performed in centres where all aspects of the disability and the vulnerability determined by the altered physiology of spinal cord injury are understood and fully catered for. Many surgical triumphs flounder and give way to unacceptable morbidity due to complications in the respiratory tract and neuropathic skin. Mutilating pressure sores have very often vitiated an otherwise highly skilful surgical undertaking, keeping the disabled person in hospital for several months with much residual deprivation of mobility and substantial reduction in the quality of life. Such a development is an outrageous negation of the philosophy of care. The most vulnerable aspect of profound physical disability is the virtual non-existence of physical and often, emotional reserve. The life of a disabled person is a delicate balance between control and decompensation. It is a balance that is achieved after great physical and emotional effort and making radical decisions affecting the direction of life will easily disturb it. Recognition of this vulnerability ought to be fundamental in any planning of treatment.

Advances in urological care have ensured that complications in the urinary tract with inevitable progression to renal insufficiency or failure are no longer common causes of death in spinal cord injured people as they were three or four decades ago (Damanski and Gibbon 1956; Tribe 1963). It is therefore unacceptable if the disabled person is denied the benefits of such advances in treatment in safety, by urological care conducted in isolation.

Use of resources for expensive and time-consuming medical treatment, however scientifically exciting, cannot be justified if the life so saved would degenerate to unacceptable social isolation, recurrent hospital admissions and ultimate confinement to an institution for the chronic sick.

References

Damanski M, Gibbon NOK (1956) The upper urinary tract in the paraplegic: a long term survey. Br J Urol 28: 24–36

Tribe GR (1963) Causes of death in the early and late stages of paraplegia. Paraplegia 1: 19–47

Chapter 2

Immediate Management of the Inability to Void

E.J. McGuire

Spinal cord injury induces a period of spinal shock during which all reflex activity below the spinal lesion is absent or markedly reduced. While reflex function is absent, internal sphincter closure is maintained and some method of bladder drainage is essential. For a number of reasons, including associated injuries requiring close monitoring of urine output, this is most frequently accomplished by Foley catheter drainage in the first 48–72 hours after injury, particularly in those patients requiring neurosurgical, orthopaedic or other surgical procedures. After initial stabilisation, the Foley catheters should be removed and intermittent catheterisation begun as soon as practicable.

Sometimes, very early after spinal cord injury, decisions are made in the name of expediency which have disastrous long-term consequences. These include the use of Foley catheters, or suprapubic tubes in patients with very high injuries, or catheter drainage used to obviate the need for very frequent catherisation in other patients. Once in place, catheters are difficult to remove until the complications of catheter drainage require that some other method of management be chosen. These complications are so difficult to manage that every effort in the early stages after spinal cord injury should be directed at avoiding the use of a catheter.

Exceptions

Elderly males who suffer spinal cord injury but have had a prior prostatectomy can be initially managed by Credé voiding rather than intermittent catherisation. In all others, Credé voiding should be avoided as internal sphincter function prevents low pressure drainage. It should be kept in mind that early assessment of the degree of completeness of an injury may be in error, and preservation of vesical reservoir capability and urethral sphincter integrity by intermittent catheterisation is the underlying goal of initial management, while waiting for the evolution of the final neural deficit.

Basic Implementation of Intermittent Catheterisation

In patients with lesions at or below T12, intermittent catheterisation is relatively easy to implement and requires no special arrangements. We monitor the volume recovered on a four hourly intermittent catheterisation schedule, and adjust the schedule to prevent volumes in excess of 600 ml. In patients with higher lesions unable to tolerate the tilt table, the same technique is used. As the spinal cord injury evolves, however, patients with cervical lesions develop peculiar urine output patterns which make it more difficult to adhere to a rigid timed schedule of intermittent catheterisation. Typically, urine output is small during the day when the patient is upright in a chair, and the interval between catheterisation can be increased. Immediately following assumption of the supine position, however, a diuresis occurs which may require hourly catheterisation. The diurnal variation becomes more prominent over time. It is generally non-productive to limit fluid intake and simply adjusting the schedule of intermittent catheterisation to compensate for a variable urine output works quite well.

Continued Intermittent Catheterisation during and after Recovery from Spinal Shock

It is perfectly practicable to continue intermittent catheterisation indefinitely in most patients with spinal cord injury (Herr 1975; McGuire and Brady 1979). However, as spinal shock dissipates, recovery of reflex activity occurs and, with time, the sphincter pressure increases in patients with suprasacral lesions as does the bladder pressure in virtually all patients with spinal cord or spinal root lesions. Because spinal shock is unpredictable and recovery of reflex activity variable, urodynamic evaluation should be periodic and begun relatively early (McGuire and Savastano 1983). The information sought from the urodynamic study is simple. Does the bladder store urine to those volumes recovered at the time of catheterisation at low pressure? Low pressure in this context is arbitrary but should be less than 20 cmH$_2$O. If so, intermittent catheterisation can be continued. If not, some method to decrease intravesical pressure is required. Sacral and infrasacral lesions (or "lower motor neurone lesions") are relatively straightforward and problems are rare, since urethral sphincter pressures are usually fixed and the bladder pressure, at the time of urinary leakage (or leak point pressure), remains relatively constant. That particular measurement is useful since it provides essential information. If leakage occurs between catheterisations, it is important to know at what pressure this occurs, since very low pressure leakage while a problem is not dangerous. On the other hand, leakage in an individual with a leak point pressure of 60 cmH$_2$O is a problem which must be treated either by reducing urethral resistance to lower the leak point pressure, or by inducing a change in bladder reservoir capability so neither leakage nor high pressures occur. In practice in patients with sacral spinal cord or root lesions, or for that matter peripheral pelvic nerve injuries, a problem with increased intravesical pressure occurs only when urethral resistance is high enough to allow it. If urethral resistance is high enough, and the bladder not emptied by intermittent catheterisation, then a dangerous elevation in intravesical pressure can occur. Alternatively, even if the bladder is emptied on a regular basis but bladder storage activity is poor, and pressure rises with volume increments high, sustained intravesical pressures can occur which are dangerous. Vesical compliance or storage of urine at low pressure can be improved with anticholinergic agents (McGuire and Savastano 1983). If sufficient capacity at low pressure cannot be achieved with anticholinergic agents (oxybutinin chloride or propantheline) then urethral resistance must be decreased, usually by sphincterotomy, or a better reservoir created by augmentation cystoplasty.

While somewhat more complex in nature, the same pressure relationships govern safe intermittent catheterisation in patients with suprasacral spinal cord lesions. In these individuals, reflex vesical activity often develops, which is frequently associated with disco-ordinate external sphincter contractility. This "detrusor-sphincter dyssynergia" can produce high sustained intravesical pressures, vesico-ureteric reflux, pyelonephritis and the other complications associated with neuropathic vesical dysfunction occurring in patients with spinal cord injury (Hackler 1977). It is, however, surprisingly easy to control detrusor contractile activity in such patients using anticholinergic agents alone, or a combination of an anticholinergic agent and a tricyclic antidepressant. There is no accurate clinical method to determine whether bladder pressures are low enough and periodic cystometrograms (CMG), with a small non-retention catheter are required to determine whether the bladder stores urine at low pressures to those volumes recovered at the time of catheterisation. If leakage between intermittent catheterisation occurs, a determination of leak point pressure is essential to plan appropriate management. For example, a 60-year-old female occasionally wet with transfers, who has a flat CMG to 600 ml and no vesical pressure rise, leaks because of relative sphincter inefficiency rather than reflex vesical contractility. While that problem is not always easily dealt with in patients with spinal cord injury, at least there is no danger to the upper urinary tract. On the other hand, a 20-year-old male paraplegic with a T6 injury leaking unpredictably between catheterisations almost certainly has reflex vesical contractility which should be identified on a CMG and the volume required to initiate the response recorded. After treatment for several days with anticholinerigic agents, the CMG should be repeated to determine storage pressures to those volumes recovered at the time of intermittent catheterisation, even if leakage no longer occurs.

Autonomic Dysreflexia and Intermittent Catheterisation

Autonomic dysreflexia is a potential problem in any patient with a lesion higher than T5 and, although rare in patients with thoracic level injuries, it is quite common in those with cervical lesions (McGuire and Rossier 1983). With regard to urinary tract function and the genesis of autonomic dysreflexia, there are two broad categories. A dysreflexic episode may be initiated by bladder volume or by bladder contractility. Usually it is difficult to tell simply by observation which of these is occurring. A CMG is helpful to determine volume tolerance, and to determine whether reflex vesical contractility is excited during the examination and with it autonomic dysreflexia. If low volume detrusor reflex contractility occurs, treatment should be directed at that entity with anticholinergic agents. If there is no reflex contractility and the dysreflexic syndrome is provoked by bladder volume only, then intermittent catheterisation schedules can be adjusted to avoid volumes associated with dysreflexia and a small dose of an alpha-blocking agent can be given to blunt the dysreflexic response (e.g. prazosin 1 mg b.i.d.). It is important to recognise that a sympathetic response to extreme bladder volumes occurs in normal man, as it does in the spinal injured population. It is the magnitude of the response which is abnormal in patients with spinal cord injury, not the response itself. In those patients with autonomic dysreflexia stimulated by bladder distension, adjustment of the catheterisation programme to include more frequent catheterisation at times of high urine output, for example, immediately after the individual returns to bed following wheelchair activities, is often all that is required.

Bacteriuria and Symptomatic Infection during the First Three Months after Spinal Cord Injury

In this patient population, bacteriuria is relatively common but symptomatic urinary tract infections are very rare. While we as yet have no good information on the effect of chronic bacteriuria in spinal cord patients managed by condom catheter drainage after sphincterotomy, or by intermittent catheterisation as a definitive method of management, we do know that if intravesical pressures are controlled within certain limits, symptomatic infection, pyelonephritis and/or urosepsis are extremely rare. In preliminary studies at the University of Michigan Medical Center at Ann Arbor during the past four years, we have been able to certainly identify symptomatic urinary infections only very rarely, and when these occur, they are often associated with a change in intravesical pressure, related to recovery of reflex function, or the development of detrusor-sphincter dyssynergia. There is a definite tendency to regard a spinal cord patient with a febrile episode as demonstrating a urinary infection. Some evidence for this is almost always found on urinalysis or urine culture. However, proof that bacteriuria in a patient chronically bacteriuric is responsible for a febrile episode, particularly when bladder pressures are found to be within normal limits, is not usually forthcoming nor do such patients show vesico-ureteric reflux, nor do they subsequently develop pyelonephritic scarring on follow-up intravenous urography. In this patient population, there is little evidence that prophylactic antimicrobial administration prevents bacteriuria, and no evidence whatsoever that prophylactic therapy ameliorates the risk of symptomatic urinary infection, or urosepsis or pyelonephritis, all of which are so rare as to be difficult to study.

Since urine cultures and urinalyses will be done, and since these patients will often become bacteriuric, treatment will inevitably be initiated. In patients with asymptomatic bacteriuria, we prefer to treat with direct instillation of an antimicrobial agent into the bladder, as, for example, a buffered solution of gentamicin (480 mg in 1 litre) instilling 30 ml of the solution into the bladder with each catheterisation. This is not absorbed, causes no harm and may have some salutary effect. This method does not mask another infectious process as can be the case with systemic antimicrobial agents.

Urinary infection in association with symptoms (i.e. fever, etc.) requires treatment with systemic antimicrobial agents, at least until some determination can be made about vesical function, storage pressure and leak point pressures. Individuals responsible for primary care of spinal cord patients usually make decisions regarding institution of antimicrobial therapy based on symptoms, and that is as it should be, since no set of rules can substitute for clinical judgement on the spot. Whether treatment was required can be decided later.

Transition from Intermittent Catheterisation as a Temporary to a Permanent Method of Management

There are two issues related to use of intermittent catheterisation (ISC) as a permanent method of management. The first is simply: is the bladder sufficiently large and of low pressure so that the technique can be used satisfactorily? The second is, can the patient, or those taking care of him, manage the technique? Patients with cervical level injuries are usually not thought capable of ISC, but a surprising number of these individuals can manage some independent intermittent catheterisation. In others, hand function is so limited that catheterisation per urethram is impossible, and provision for a continent abdominal stoma constructed from bladder, small bowel, or as part of an augmentation cystoplasty can be made (Steinberg et al. 1987). This can make life easier for patients and attendants in very high quadriplegics with no hand function as well. Patients should be taught a clean technique, rather than sterile technique, a departure from the rigid asepsis practised by the catheterisation team in hospitalised patients.

Alternative Methods

An alternative to intermittent catheterisation is clearly required in some patients whose bladder pressure cannot be controlled, or for whom the technique itself is physically impossible. In males, particularly those with high injuries, reflex vesical activity is rarely sufficiently long in duration to induce adequate vesical emptying. Total sphincterotomy including both the internal and external sphincter is a reasonable method of management. Before this is done, a determination as to whether a condom catheter can be worn is required. Following sphincterotomy, urodynamic evaluation should be repeated periodically to be certain that leak point pressures remain below 20 cmH$_2$O. Leak point pressures are a reliable measure of the effect of a sphincterotomy or any sphincter ablative procedure. If leak point pressures are very low (10–15 cmH$_2$O) Credé voiding can be used to ensure more complete bladder emptying. Problems related to penile size and girth in patients wearing condom catheters, troubled by reflex erectile activity during condom application, with subsequent loss of condom adhesion can often be treated by implantation of the smallest diameter penile prosthesis available.

In females, continence is of overriding importance, and leakage related to detrusor compliance, or reflex activity which cannot be controlled with medication may require augmentation cystoplasty. Incontinence related to poor sphincter function, in the presence of adequate bladder capacity, can be treated by an appropriate surgical procedure on the urethra, usually a pubovaginal sling (McGuire et al. 1987). Increases in sphincteric resistance attained by surgical procedures can induce detrusor hyperreflexia, or diminished vesical compliance, and routine urodynamic testing is required on a regular basis after such procedures to be certain that intravesical pressures remain low.

References

Hackler RH (1977) A 25-year prospective mortality study in the spinal cord injured patient: comparision with the long term living paraplegic. J Urol 117: 486–488

Herr HW (1975) Intermittent catheterization in neurogenic bladder dysfunction. J Urol 113: 477–479

McGuire EJ, Brady S (1979) Detrusor sphincter dyssynergia. J Urol 121: 774–777

McGuire EJ, Rossier AB (1983) Treatment of acute autonomic dysreflexia. J Urol 129: 1185–1186.

McGuire EJ, Savastano JA (1983) Long term follow-up of spinal cord injury patients managed by intermittent catheterization. J Urol 129: 775–776

McGuire EJ, Bennett CJ, Konnack JA, Sonda LP, Savastano JA, (1987) experience with pubovaginal slings for urinary incontinence at the University of Michigan. J Urol 138: 525–526

Steinberg R, Bennett C, Konnack J, Savastano J, McGuire E (1987) Construction of a low pressure reservoir and achievement of continence after "diversion" and in end stage vesical dysfunction. J Urol 138: 39–41

Chapter 3

A Practical Approach to Urodynamic Evaluation

D.R. Staskin and R.J. Krane

Introduction

The management of the lower urinary tract following spinal cord injury is a high priority for both the patient and physician. The major concerns are the preservation of renal function, the selection of a safe and convenient treatment alternative for the management of urinary storage and emptying, and the institution of a practical daily regimen which may prevent the commonly observed sequelae associated with lower urinary tract dysfunction following spinal cord injury.

The most serious concern is the preservation of renal function. Hydronephrosis, pyelonephritis, and renal lithiasis are the primary causes of renal scarring, loss of functioning renal parenchyma, and renal failure. Lower urinary tract dysfunction is commonly implicated in the development of these forms of upper tract disease, especially when characterised by the findings of recurrent urinary tract infections, elevated post-micturition residual urine, chronically elevated intravesical pressure and vesico-ureteric reflux.

Efficient lower urinary tract function is a product of the dynamic interaction of the two functional areas of the lower urinary tract, the detrusor and sphincteric mechanisms whose reflex behaviour is normally modulated by cerebral control. A low pressure reservoir with adequate outlet resistance is required for continence, while a well sustained detrusor contraction in the absence of obstruction is required for efficient emptying. Lower urinary tract management following spinal cord injury often involves the choice between facilitating storage or improving emptying, one often to the detriment of the other. Regardless of the choice, a knowledge of the individual and integrated behaviour of the bladder and bladder outlet which can be obtained from urodynamic evaluation is required.

The increased ability to describe accurately voiding dynamics in the spinal cord injury patient has led to an improved understanding of the normal and abnormal function of the detrusor and the sphincteric mechanisms. Urodynamic studies have also provided objective information which has proved useful for classifying the behaviour of the bladder and bladder outlet and for instituting therapy. Although current urodynamic techniques have not allowed accurate prospective identification of individuals at risk for upper tract deterioration, several groups of patients with similar neurological lesions and detrusor and sphincter behaviour have been identified to be at higher risk. In addition, urodynamic evaluation has improved the ability to select therapy which addresses the underlying pathophysiology in patients with established or progressive upper tract disease.

Neuro-urological Classification and Urodynamic Techniques: an Historical Approach

The Physical Examination

The early descriptions of voiding dysfunction in patients with spinal cord injury were determined by the findings on neurological examination. By the early 1900s, the "reflex", "automatic" (Muller 1902) or "normal" cord bladder characterised by a preserved micturition reflex had been differentiated from the autonomous (Munro 1937) or autonomic (Slater 1954) bladder associated with an absence of reflex contractility. The importance of identifying the location of the lesion above or below the level of the sacral micturition nuclei in determining the type of lower urinary tract dysfunction was widely accepted by the 1950s (Giertz and Lindbloom 1951).

Bors and Comarr (1971) classified neurological lesions as either upper or lower motor neurone with respect to the anatomical relationship of the injury to the sacral cord reflex centres. An upper motor neurone lesion presumed involvement of the descending suprasacral autonomic pathways to the bladder and somatic pathways to the lower extremities. In this classification, suprasacral spinal cord lesions would be expected to result in reflex spasticity of the bladder and the lower extremities. A lower motor neurone lesion involving pre- and postganglionic fibres to the bladder and the somatic nerves to the lower extremities would be expected to produce vesical (visceromotor–bladder) and lower extremity (somatomotor) flaccidity. A "mixed" lesion group accounts for the exceptions: lower extremity spasticity and an areflexic bladder, and normal or flaccid lower extremities with a hyperreflexic bladder.

Unfortunately, neurological examination alone is insufficient in classifying bladder behaviour following spinal cord injury, especially in those patients with paraplegia who present with spinal column lesions from T10 to L2. The urological presentation may vary after injury to the reflex micturition nuclei and the somatic nuclei in the conus medullaris and the peripheral nerves depending on individual anatomy and the type of the lesion. In addition, lesions of the conus medullaris, or segments immediately above this level may result in a mixed neurological presentation secondary to direct injury to the sacral cord or descending cord infarction. The presence of "spinal shock" may also produce a sacral–infrasacral rather than a suprasacral presentation for up to nine months following the injury.

Post-Void Residual Urine

Bors and Comarr (1971) included a measurement of the post-void residual urine determination (PVR) in addition to the physical examination in their classification of voiding dysfunction following spinal cord injury. In the Bors-Comarr classification, voiding efficiency is expressed as the percentage of the ratio of residual urine to bladder capacity. An "unbalanced bladder" indicated the presence of greater than 20% of the total bladder capacity in residual urine in a patient with an upper motor neurone lesion and 10% in a patient with a lower motor neurone lesion.

Unfortunately, using the physical examination and the criteria for a "balanced bladder", one cannot differentiate several significantly different voiding patterns. An elevated residual urine in a suprasacral lesion may imply a non-contractile bladder, insufficient reflex bladder contractility or detrusor-sphincter dyssynergia. In an infrasacral lesion, the inability to produce significant abdominal straining or the inability to overcome outlet resistance may also produce elevated residual urine. Of even greater prognostic concern, however, is the inability of the PVR measurement to reflect intravesical pressure during voiding or during urinary storage between voiding episodes. A low PVR alone, although helpful in indicating the ability to empty, should not be accepted as a criterion for predicting future lower or upper urinary tract status. The attempt to simplify and classify voiding behaviour by examination and PVR alone should not be interpreted as the only approach to voiding dysfunction described by Bors and Comarr, as is seen in their detailed review of urodynamic techniques (Bors 1957).

Cystometry

Due to the failure of the physical examination, and the residual urine volume determination adequately to describe voiding dysfunction, cystometry was applied to the evaluation of spinal cord injury patients. Cystometric correlation of bladder behaviour with the somatic conditions of spasticity and flaccidity was reported in 1940 by Voris and Landes (1940). Lapides (1976) popularised the description of the cystometric (capacity, proprioception, contractility, heat and cold sensation, residual urine) findings associated with many types of neuropathic voiding dysfunction. The Lapides system created five categories based on the objective measurement of bladder function by cystometry, urinary residual and bladder sensation (Table 3.1)

Table 3.1. Lapides cystometric classification of the neuropathic bladder

Reflex neuropathic bladder
Sensory neuropathic bladder
Motor paralytic bladder
Autonomous neuropathic bladder
Uninhibited neuropathic bladder

Suprasacral lesions are represented by the "reflex" and "uninhibited" neuro-pathic bladder. The reflex neuropathic bladder is most commonly used to describe the complete interruption of the spinal pathways between the brainstem and sacral micturition centre. There is an absence of bladder sensation and hyperreflexic bladder contractions are present without voluntary micturition. The potential for increased urinary residual volumes and the development of decreased bladder compliance differentiate this category from the uninhibited bladder which is presumed to result from injury or disease in the "corticoregulatory tract", which has an inhibitory effect on micturition. In the "uninhibited bladder" voluntary contraction of the bladder is possible, sensation is intact, and residual urine is small. This situation occurs rarely in spinal cord injury patients and implies an incomplete lesion, which had spared both the sensory tracts and the tracts which co-ordinate detrusor and sphincter function. Any classification of voiding dysfunction in spinal injury patients based on the cystometric curves alone fails to provide critical information concerning outlet function.

Cystometry has been considered the reflex hammer of the neuro-urologist, (Nesbit and Baum 1954) and may be performed by various techniques. The most common variations involve the filling medium (gas, water, or radiographic contrast), the filling rate (patient's own urine production ranging up to 125 ml per minute), and the access to the bladder (per urethram or suprapubic).

The type of information which is required may determine the type of cystometry which is most efficient and practical. If the purpose of the study is merely to identify the presence or absence of reflex bladder contractility by eliciting an isometric bladder contraction, the study can be performed with carbon dioxide at a fast filling rate through a Foley catheter. If a more accurate deter-mination of bladder compliance and bladder capacity is desired, a more physio-logical filling rate which approaches the patient's normal urine production is required.

Cystometry performed to evaluate bladder emptying requires the use of fluid and a catheterisation technique which does not provide significant obstruction to flow. The amount of artefactual resistance provided by the catheter is directly related to both the size of the catheter and the degree of obstruction. The 8 or 10 French double lumen catheter which is commercially available for multichannel voiding studies is usually adequate in patients without significant obstruction, but many patients with significant outlet obstruction secondary to detrusor-sphincter dyssynergia, who are able to void outside the testing situation, may be unable to void around this catheter. Suprapubic catheter placement may be necessary if accurate pressure-flow information is desirable. Extreme care should be taken to assure a sterile urine before using this technique because of possible urinary extravasation into the retropubic space at the time of placement, during the study and after suprapubic catheter removal.

Simple Cystometry

The cystometric curve in the absence of a detrusor contraction may be divided into three segments:

1. the initial pressure rise (0–5 cmH$_2$O) representing the initial viscoelastic response of the bladder and active contraction of the detrusor

2. the tonus limb (normally flat) representing the accommodation of increasing volume at a constant pressure and the compliance of the connective tissue elements of the bladder
3. the terminal segment (increasing pressure) representing the elastic limits of collagen and elastic components of the bladder.

Conditions associated with fibrosis have been demonstrated to cause an increase in the tonus limb, the second portion of the curve. Although parasympathetic denervation has been associated with decreased bladder compliance, several investigators have proposed that the major factor leading to loss of compliance is collagen deposition and is not a response to denervation (Tang and Ruch 1955; Klevmark 1977). Others have suggested a contribution from a change in the neuromuscular receptor response, from a beta-relaxation response to an alpha-adrenergic contractile response to sympathetic stimulation, which effects detrusor smooth muscle relaxation during bladder filling (Sundin et al. 1977).

The shape of the cystometric curve may also be influenced by rapid bladder filling. If normal compliance is demonstrated, the filling rate is less critical. However, fast-fill cystometry may elicit low bladder compliance (intravesical pressure observed at a selected bladder volume during filling) which is demonstrated during cystometry but may not be reproduced at the rate of the patient's urinary production. When a low compliant bladder is demonstrated during rapid-fill cystometry, the filling rate should be noted and the study should be repeated at a more physiological filling rate before a clinical diagnosis is established. A simple method for confirming that a portion of the low compliance may not be reproduced at a more natural filling rate is to continue the intravesical pressure monitoring at the established volume after the inflow has been stopped. The intravesical pressure will slowly decline to a level which better approximates the intravesical pressure which exists during physiological filling; however, it may not return to the true baseline (Coolsaet et al. 1973).

The filling rate has also been shown to affect the volume and pressure at which a reflex bladder contraction can be provoked. Fast-fill cystometry will often elicit a reflex bladder contraction at an intravesical volume less than the true bladder capacity.

We have found the measurement of concomitant intra-abdominal pressure with a rectal catheter to be of limited use in the evaluation of patients with suprasacral lesions, since the contribution of intra-abdominal pressure is usually negligible. In sacral-infrasacral lesions, where the abdominal musculature is preserved and patients are required to void by abdominal straining, the technique is useful for confirming this voiding pattern.

Pharmacological Testing

Bethanechol Supersensitivity Test

Based upon Cannon's findings that a denervated organ becomes supersensitive to a neurohumoral transmitter, Lapides et al. (1962) reported a test for the diagnosis of detrusor denervation. Fluid cystometry at a filling rate of 60 ml per minute is performed to a volume of 100 ml to establish the baseline. Bethanechol chloride at a dose of 2.5 mg is given subcutaneously and cystometry is repeated at 10, 20 and 30 minutes post injection. An intravesical pressure rise of greater than 15 cmH_2O was established as a positive test for denervation. The bethanechol test has been accepted as a means of distinguishing neuropathic from non-neuropathic causes of the non-contractile detrusor, but not without modifications of the technique, and questions concerning its accuracy (Fig. 3.1).

The test has been modified by the use of gas (Merrill and Rotta 1983), by using 5.0 mg of bethanechol (Pavlakis et al. 1983) and by pre-filling the bladder to 100 ml and, after injection, performing constant monitoring at this volume while utilising 20 cmH_2O elevation as the pressure rise indicative of neuropathy (Glahn 1970).

False positive results have been attributed to cystitis, emotional stress, and rapid diuresis during the monitoring period. These can be avoided in the spinal injury patient by ensuring a sterile urine and monitoring the output at the termination of the study. False negative results have been attributed to myogenic failure, poor absorption of the bethanechol in extremely obese patients, and time of the study which may not be positive until up to six months following the injury. Although false positive results have been reported in up to 50% and false negative results in up to 26% of patients in one reported series (Blaivas et al. 1980) this particular study was performed in a group of patients who were selected because of an acontractile bladder on cystometry and whose diagnosis was equivocal for lower motor neurone lesions after careful neurological diagnosis and myelography. In those patients whose neurological diagnosis was established by an abnormal electromyogram, no false positives and 2% false negatives were noted. It is evident that the patient population which is tested and the method of establishing the diagnosis may influence the accuracy in confirming the diagnosis of a neuropathic lesion.

The bethanechol test has been suggested for use in testing the therapeutic efficacy of the drug in promoting micturition. Clinical studies have demonstrated the need for intact sacral reflex pathways for the drug to be effective (Downie et al. 1983); no correlation between a positive test and improved micturition (Wein et al. 1980); and evidence that bethanechol enhances the obstructive effects of the urethra in patients with spinal cord injury (Yalla and Gittes 1977).

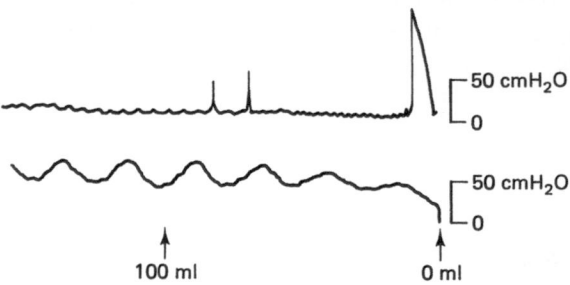

Figure 3.1 Bethanechol sensitivity test (BST). Upper cystogram illustrates detrusor areflexia. At a volume of 100 ml, intravesical pressure is 10 cmH_2O. Lower tracing was recorded approximately 15 minutes after 5 mg bethanechol hydrochloride was injected subcutaneously. At 100 ml volume, intravesical pressure has risen to about 50 cmH_2O. This represents positive BST.

Extended Voiding Cystometry

In addition to the rate-dependent decrease in compliance and the non-physiological provocation of detrusor contractions, fast-fill simple cystometry does not allow an accurate measurement of the duration or frequency of bladder contractions which are stimulated by physiological filling rates. We have used extended voiding cystometry in our institution in order to document the frequency, amplitude and duration of bladder contractions as well as the intravesical pressure which remains between bladder contractions. Analysis of these parameters also allows the calculation of the percentage of time in which the patient develops and maintains elevated intravesical pressures during normal voiding cycles. The suprasacral spinal cord patients who were evaluated demonstrated frequent (2.1 contractions/hour), high-amplitude (56.8 cmH$_2$O), long-duration contractions (4.0 minutes/contraction), and had substantial time (13.8% of time monitored) with contractile activity which maintained intravesical pressures greater than 40 cmH$_2$O (8.4%), but had experienced no evidence of upper tract disease. Five patients with upper tract changes who underwent extended voiding cystometry demonstrated increasing bladder pressure between contractions as the residual urine increased (poor bladder compliance) and had an intravesical pressure greater than 40 cmH$_2$O for more than 47% of the time monitored (Staskin et al. 1988) (Table 3.2).

The parameters of contraction frequency and duration and the pressure of the residual urine (when not emptied by intermittent catheterisation) may be useful in identifying contractility patterns which predispose to upper tract disease and help to establish criteria for therapeutic intervention prior to the development of upper urinary tract changes.

Krane and Siroky (1979) incorporated the urodynamic information available from combined studies of the detrusor (cystometry) and external sphincter (electromyography) into a scheme which provided an objective description of neuropathic voiding dysfunction. The abnormalities of detrusor control (hyperreflexia, normoreflexia, or areflexia) and sphincter function (dyssynergia or non-relaxation) can be measured objectively and categorised by urodynamic testing (Table 3.3).

Patients with detrusor hyperreflexia and co-ordinated sphincter activity are expected to have low post-void residual urine, absence of high-pressure voiding, and an absence of upper urinary tract deterioration and can be managed with anticholinergic medication with or without intermittent catheterisation or a collection device.

Table 3.2. Results of extended voided cystometry

Results	Normal upper tracts			Hydroureteronephrosis
n	20			5
F = (contractions/hour)	mean 2.2	(0.6–4.0)	P 0.01*	4.6 (4.5–4.7)
D = (minutes/contraction)	mean 5.0	(1.2–30.3)	ns	2.4 (1.8–3.5)
A = (cmH$_2$O)	mean 57.8	(22–100)	ns	32.7 (20–46)
%C = (minutes contracting/total)	mean 14.6	(1–45)	ns	15.8 (14–19)
%P40 = (press 40 cm/total)	mean 10.2	(2–25)	P 0.05*	47.8 (27–78)
ICP = (cmH$_2$O)	mean 3.3	(0–14)	P 0.01*	38.0 (36–48)

* Statistically significant.

Table 3.3. Categories of sphincteric activity with a contractile bladder or an acontractile bladder

---

Detrusor hyperreflexia (or normoreflexia)
  Co-ordinated sphincters
  Striated-sphincter dyssynergia
  Smooth-muscle sphincter dyssynergia
  Non-relaxing smooth-muscle sphincter

Detrusor areflexia
  Co-ordinated sphincters
  Non-relaxing striated sphincter
  Denervated striated sphincter
  Non-relaxing smooth-muscle sphincter

Patients with detrusor hyperreflexia and vesicosphincter dyssynergia will usually present with evidence of outflow obstruction, including increased detrusor contraction pressures, poor flow and an elevated post-void residual urine. Upper tract deterioration may result from acquired reflux, or chronically elevated intravesical pressure and detrusor hypertrophy resulting in obstruction of the intramural ureter. Therapy which is orientated towards the bladder involves conversion of the hyperreflexia and poor compliance by pharmacological (anticholinergics) or surgical (augmentation) means. Alternatively, therapy for the sphincter involves sphincterotomy, or bypassing the sphincter by permanent or intermittent catheterisation.

Detrusor hyperreflexia and dyssynergia of the proximal smooth muscle sphincter is seen almost exclusively in patients with upper cord lesions and associated autonomic dysreflexia. This is often accompanied by skeletal muscle dyssynergia. Pharmacological therapy uses alpha-adrenergic and skeletal muscle antagonists. Transurethral resection of the bladder neck (smooth muscle) in addition to external sphincterotomy (skeletal muscle) should be considered.

Detrusor areflexia with a co-ordinated sphincter is seen in patients with a sacral or infrasacral lesion. Treatment is Credé's emptying of the bladder or intermittent catheterisation.

Detrusor areflexia with evidence of external sphincter denervation is observed with injury to the parasympathetic and pudendal nerve outflows and is associated with sacral or infrasacral injury. These patients will present with incontinence and a paradoxically increased residual urine volume. Intermittent catheterisation will suffice in males who will remain continent if the bladder neck and prostate are intact. In females with resultant stress incontinence from a combination of levator and urethral denervation, a urethral suspension or sling procedure is often necessary in combination with intermittent catheterisation. The other combinations of detrusor and sphincter function are clinically rare.

Urodynamic studies of varying levels of sophistication are necessary. Often this involves only a cystometrogram and electromyogram, but videourodynamic studies are necessary for the evaluation of bladder neck function.

Electromyographic Recording

Electromyography of the pelvic floor may vary in the type of electrode (coaxial or monopolar needle or external patch surface electrodes), the site which is selected (external anal sphincter, periurethral sphincter or levator musculature), the type of signal (individual motor potential or gross muscle group activity), and the method of recording (audiographic, strip chart recording, or oscilloscopic tracing). Both the integrity of innervation and the kinetics of sphincter function can be assessed depending on the choice.

Surface electrodes usually consist of a metallic contact incorporated within a patch which is placed on the perineal or perianal skin. Other contact positions may be obtained by incorporation into a urethral catheter (Nordling et al. 1978), an anal plug (Bradley et al. 1975) or a vaginal tampon (Kiesswett 1976). Problems with placement and adherence are common, especially in female patients. Studies are limited to gross measurements of muscle group activity. The net integrated activity of the muscle groups and, occasionally, activity from undesired groups, is displayed on a chart recorder.

Needle electrodes placed intramuscularly may be bipolar-coaxial-concentric (central core with surrounding outer needle with potentials measured between the two) or monopolar which requires a second electrode, often a patch electrode, to act as the reference. The monopolar needles have been produced as wire electrodes which are placed through an introducer and tend to be smaller and less traumatic for patients who have intact sensation.

Although the morphology and innervation of the external anal sphincter, levator musculature, external intrinsic urethral sphincter, and external urethral sphincter are different the results are usually clinically comparable unless partial peripheral denervation is present. For anal electromyography the needle is placed at the mucocutaneous junction. Urethral sphincter electromyography is performed in male patients by insertion of the needle electrode in the midline between the anus and the posterior scrotum towards the apex of the prostate. The needle will traverse the bulbospongiosus muscle and then the external urethral sphincter. Resting activity may not be demonstrated but needle placement may be confirmed by tugging on a urethral catheter, or by squeezing the tip of the penis (bulbocavernosus reflex). In female patients, urethral sphincter studies require electrode insertion in a midline and ventral direction above the urethra.

In patients without a neurological lesion, baseline activity represents the firing of individual motor units. The recruitment of additional activity can be observed with voluntary contraction; Credé manoeuvre; cough; glans or clitoral stimulation; or bladder filling (guarding reflex) (Fig. 3.2). Decreased sphincter activity is noted prior to bladder contraction and the electromyogram (EMG) remains silent during detrusor activity (Fig. 3.3).

Upper motor neurone lesions classically spare the anterior horn cell and peripheral nerve. All of the reflexes remain intact, but voluntary control may be absent. Depending on the completeness of the lesion, unco-ordinated voiding or detrusor sphincter dyssynergia may be noted (Fig. 3.4). A spinal cord lesion is necessary for this diagnosis and the finding of increased EMG activity secondary to voluntary tightening in order to prevent urinary loss, straining, or failure to relax the pelvic floor during voiding should not be confused with vesicosphincter dyssynergia. Another common misinterpretation is to see increased sphincter activity with filling in a bladder with poor compliance and to assume that the detrusor pressure represents a bladder contraction. An involuntary bladder contraction with an involuntary increase in sphincter activity is required for the diagnosis of detrusor sphincter dyssynergia. Dyssynergic activity has been divided into subgroups depending on its temporal relationship to the detrusor contraction, but these patterns have not yet been shown to be of specific diagnostic or prognostic significance (Blaivas et al. 1979; Siroky and Krane, 1982; Yalla and Gittes, 1977).

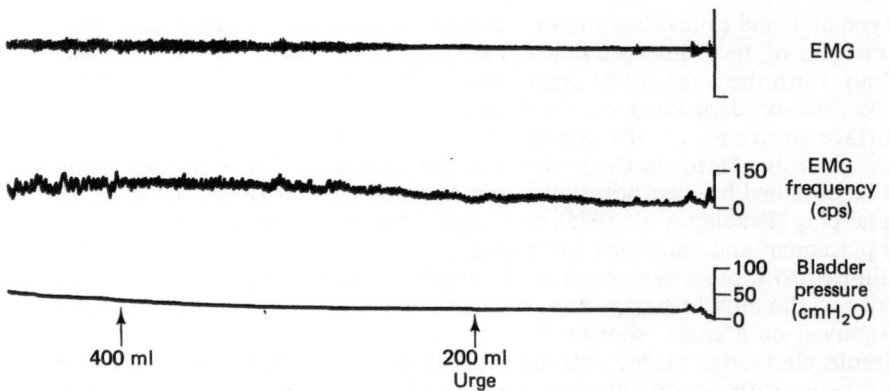

Figure 3.2 Combined cystometry and pelvic floor electromyography showing normal interaction between bladder and external sphincter. Immediately before voiding contraction, relaxation begins to occur in striated pelvic floor.

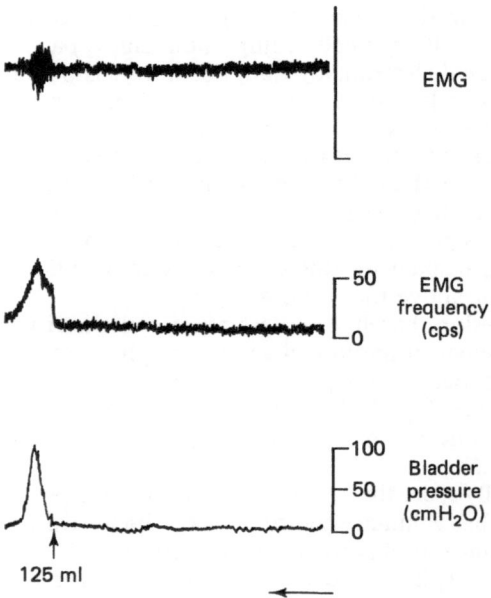

Figure 3.3 Vesicosphincter dyssynergia demonstrated by combined cystometric and pelvic floor electromyographic study. During uninhibited bladder contraction, which occurs at approximately 130 ml of intravesical volume, there is inappropriate firing of striated sphincter. Guarding, which is usually characteristic of patients with sphincter dyssynergia and complete spinal cord injury, is absent.

Lower Motor Neurone Lesions

With complete lower motor neurone lesions there is loss of both motor and sensory function to the sphincteric area. Correlation with detrusor function depends on the location and nature of the lesion. Immediately after a complete

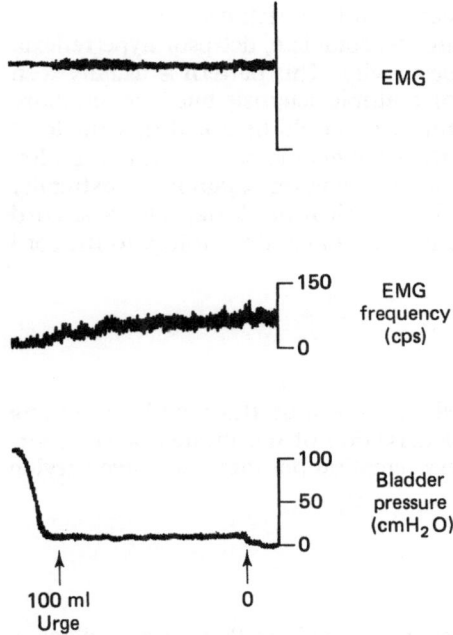

EMG

EMG frequency (cps)

Bladder pressure (cmH₂O)

100 ml
Urge

0

Figure 3.4 Combined cystometry and electromyographic study demonstrating detrusor hyperreflexia with appropriate relaxation of striated sphincter. This pattern of interaction is seen in patients with suprapontine lesions and incomplete suprasacral cord lesions.

lesion there is a loss of both voluntary and reflex activity for up to six weeks. Polyphasic potentials (more than four deflections on an oscilloscopic tracing) denote partial reinnervation which is characterised by incomplete reflex activity and poor recruitment with voluntary contraction. Fibrillations (short duration bi- or triphasic waves) and positive sharp waves (biphasic wave with minimal negative deflection) are associated with complete denervation.

The use of combined cystometry and sphincter electromyography as opposed to cystometry alone produces better appreciation of abnormal voiding patterns in patients with spinal cord injury. In the normal individual, electromyographic activity increases with increasing bladder filling. This has been characterised as the guarding reflex. During bladder emptying a normal inhibitable bladder contraction will occur only after relaxation of the smooth and striated sphincters. The neurological integration of sphincter and bladder activity is co-ordinated at the pontine level. This area is mediated by higher cerebral centres in order to allow this long-routed reflex to occur. Contractility of the bladder is preserved following suprasacral cord injuries since the afferent and efferent nerves between the bladder and sacral cord remain intact, but detrusor-sphincter co-ordination may be absent (vesico-sphincter dyssynergia). Because of the potential to develop chronically elevated intravesical pressures this group of patients is most likely to develop upper tract and renal decompensation.

In sacral-infrasacral lesions the detrusor pattern is one of areflexia with or without sphincter denervation. In this group of patients intravesical storage pressures usually remain low, unless a decrease in bladder compliance develops, due to decreased bladder activity or decreased outlet resistance.

In patients with spinal cord lesions that are less complete, detrusor hyperreflexia may be present with co-ordinated sphincter activity. This pattern is usually seen in patients with spinal cord involvement of multiple sclerosis but is much more uncommon in patients with spinal cord injury. It should be noted that the level of the spinal cord injury need not dictate the urodynamic pattern which results. A number of patients with cervical cord trauma may never regain lower extremity or bladder reflexes and may continue to have vesical areflexia. Thoracic cord lesions may also exhibit vesical areflexia because of longitudinal injury to the cord or vascular injury to the distal cord.

Sacral Lesions

Patients with sacral lesions will usually exhibit vesical areflexia and, depending on the extent of the injury, concomitant denervation of the striated pelvic floor. These patients will usually present in urinary retention but may also have varying degrees of incontinence.

Spinal Shock

The term spinal shock has been used to describe a condition that results following injury to the spinal cord in that there is a depression of neural activity and reflex activity below the level of the lesion. The return of flexor and extensor reflex responses of the lower extremities usually heralds the end of the spinal shock phase. It is of interest that reflexes of the very distal spinal cord (e.g. bulbocavernosus reflex) usually return almost immediately while lower extremity reflexes often take months to reappear.

Functional Classification of Voiding Dysfunction

Wein (1981) classified voiding dysfunction by using a functional approach which is orientated toward the storage and emptying functions of the lower urinary tract and the behaviour of its components, the bladder and outlet. We have modified this classification and combined it with many of the categories of the Krane and Siroky classification, using terminology instituted by the International Continence Society (Bates et al. 1981) for diagnostic use in our urodynamic laboratory. The classification is also useful for determining lower urinary tract therapy following spinal cord injury (Table 3.4).

Functional Approach to Urodynamics in the Spinal Cord Patient

Urodynamic studies can be used to describe objectively the parameters of bladder and outlet function following spinal cord injury and can be used to identify a subgroup of patients who are at greater risk for upper tract deterioration and to select the appropriate therapeutic intervention or evaluate the results of previous

Table 3.4. Functional classification of bladder and outlet activity following spinal cord injury

Incontinence

Overactive bladder (increased intravesical pressure)
    Detrusor hyperreflexia
    Decreased detrusor compliance
    Overflow incontinence (normal compliance with elevated pressure secondary to a competent
    bladder outlet)

Underactive outlet (decreased outlet resistance)
    Denervated bladder neck-proximal urethra
    Denervated external sphincter
    Iatrogenic (e.g. sphincterotomy, chronic catheter drainage)

Urinary retention

Underactive bladder (decreased intravesical pressure)
    Poorly sustained detrusor contraction
    Non-contractile bladder
        Neuropathic
        Myogenic
        Pharmacological (anticholinergic therapy)

Overactive outlet (increased outlet resistance)
    Smooth sphincter dyssynergia
    Striated sphincter dyssynergia
    Concomitant urologic disease (e.g. prostatic obstruction)
    Iatrogenic (e.g. external clamp, artificial sphincter, perineal compression)

Combined bladder and/or outlet dysfunction (mixed abnormalities)
    Overactive bladder and overactive outlet (± incontinence and ± residual)
    (e.g. detrusor hyperreflexia with sphincter dyssynergia; detrusor hyperreflexia or low
    compliance with artificial sphincter)
    Underactive bladder and underactive outlet (± incontinence and ± residual)
    (e.g. detrusor and sphincter denervation)
    Overactive bladder and underactive outlet (± incontinence and low residual)
    (e.g. detrusor hyperreflexia/post sphincterotomy)
    Underactive bladder and overactive outlet (± incontinence and high residuals)
    (e.g. detrusor areflexia with elevated leak pressure)

therapy aimed at improving urinary storage or bladder emptying. Insight into the role of lower urinary tract dysfunction in the aetiology of recurrent urinary tract infections and the symptoms of autonomic dysreflexia may also be gained. The primary goal of urodynamic studies in spinal injury patients should be to identify patients at high risk from upper tract changes secondary to chronically elevated intravesical pressure. Chronic elevation of intravesical pressure above 40 cmH$_2$O may result in functional obstruction of the upper urinary tract at the level of the uretero-vesical junction and upper tract changes even in the absence of vesico-ureteric reflux. The sequelae of bladder denervation in patients with infrasacral lesions and prolonged outlet obstruction in patients with suprasacral lesions are detrusor hypertrophy, collagen deposition within the detrusor musculature, and decreased detrusor compliance. Therefore, patients with an *overactive bladder* (detrusor hyperreflexia or low bladder compliance), particularly if they maintain an *elevated residual urine pressure* (greater than 40 cmH$_2$O), should be placed within a risk group. Urinary storage is a product of the interaction of the bladder and bladder outlet. Chronic outlet obstruction is generally recognised as a predisposing factor to upper tract changes, as a result of increased voiding pressures during bladder emptying. However, the importance of bladder outlet competence during storage, which allows the overactive bladder to maintain residual urine at chronically elevated pressures without permitting urinary leakage (*leak* pressure greater than 40 cmH$_2$O) may be an equally or more important contributing factor to the underlying pathophysiology of upper tract obstruction.

Urodynamic Studies at Initial Presentation

All spinal cord injury patients after the spinal shock phase undergo a video-urodynamic evaluation (Table 3.5) and an upper tract evaluation. This initial study is performed in order to categorise patients with respect to their potential to develop upper tract changes. The patients at high risk are identified by the presence of obstructive flow patterns, increased residual urine, elevated intravesical pressure at rest and during voiding, loss of detrusor sphincter co-ordination, or vesico-ureteric reflux. Therapy to decrease intravesical pressure after this initial evaluation is usually reserved for patients exhibiting vesico-ureteric reflux, elevated detrusor pressure during voiding (greater than 90 cmH$_2$O) or autonomic dysreflexia.

Longitudinal Urodynamic Studies

After the initial evaluation, all patients are re-evaluated yearly by the same urodynamic protocol. Patients at high risk for upper tract deterioration may exhibit increased residual urine volume, increased post-voiding intravesical pressure reflecting loss of bladder compliance, increased outlet resistance, or the development of vesico-ureteric reflux. The ability to identify patients who require attention for the combination of bladder overactivity and normal or overactive sphincteric function is improved with urodynamic evaluation. Low intravesical pressure should be maintained during and, more importantly, between detrusor contractions. This can be accomplished by treatment which suppresses frequent, long-duration, high-amplitude detrusor contractions in the presence of outlet obstruction. The appropriate therapy may involve the institution of anticholinergic therapy or augmentation of the bladder with bowel, the relief of obstructive voiding patterns by improving emptying with intermittent catheterisation, or sphincterotomy. Patients who present with and maintain a compliant bladder, who void with low intravesical pressure due to the absence or prior relief of obstruction, or who leak at low intravesical pressure are expected to be less prone to upper tract deterioration.

Table 3.5. Urodynamic evaluation

Non-invasive urinary flow rate determination
   Resting pressure of residual urine (opening pressure)
   Post-void residual urine volume
   Filling cystometry
   Simultaneous pressure-flow-EMG-VCUG

Urodynamic Evaluation for Incontinence in Spinal Cord Injury Patients

Urinary continence requires a competent bladder outlet, and a bladder which stores urine at a low intravesical pressure. The presence of a compliant bladder and the absence of uninhibited bladder contractions are necessary in order to maintain a low intravesical pressure. Therapy in order to achieve continence may involve decreasing bladder activity or increasing outlet resistance. Therapy which improves continence by increasing outlet resistance in the presence of an overactive bladder is specifically contraindicated because of the risk of upper tract deterioration.

Urodynamic Evaluation for Recurrent Urinary Tract Infection

Bladder emptying requires a detrusor contraction of sufficient force and duration (or transmission of intra-abdominal pressure to the bladder by Credé) accompanied by a co-ordinated lowering of outlet resistance at the level of the bladder neck, prostatic urethra and external sphincter. A decrease in the neurogenic facilitation (cerebral, pontine and intraspinal pathways) of the detrusor, or myogenic failure in the presence or absence of outlet obstruction may result in poor bladder emptying. Many patients referred for urodynamic evaluation because of recurrent urinary tract infection are noted to have a high residual urine volume. A common assumption is that there is underlying outlet obstruction, despite the fact that many of these patients have undergone prior external sphincterotomy. Often the failure to empty the bladder completely is due to the bladder, rather than that the outlet and repeat sphincterotomy is not expected to be successful.

The use of a pressure/flow examination with voiding cystography is useful for establishing the presence and location of outlet obstruction in these patients. Many patients with lesions above the thoracic outflow have had prior external sphincterotomy but have not had transurethral incision or resection of the bladder neck. The fluoroscopic study allows identification of the level of obstruction and when performed with voiding cystometry allows observation of the pressure required to open the bladder neck area.

Current urodynamic techniques when applied in a logical and practical manner have been instrumental in developing and applying treatment options by providing objective information concerning bladder and outlet function. The application of newer techniques such as extended voiding cystometry and the appreciation of additional factors such as post-voiding residual urine pressure, which reflects the development of poor bladder compliance and recognises the significance of prolonged intravesical storage pressure, may permit identification of patients who are at greater risk for the development of upper tract dysfunction. Therapy to manage incontinence or to improve or attain continence also requires the recognition of dynamic interaction of the bladder and bladder outlet and the contribution that can be made by careful urodynamic assessment.

References

Bates CP, Bradley WE, Glen H et al. (1981) Terminology related to neuromuscular dysfunction of
    the lower urinary tract. Br J Urol 53: 330–335
Blaivas JG, Sinha HP, Zayed AAH, Labib K (1979) Detrusor sphincter dyssynergia. J Urol 121: 774
Blaivas JG, Labib KB, Michalik SJ, Zayed AAH (1980) Failure of bethanechol denervation supersen-
    sitivity as a diagnostic aid. J Urol 123: 199–201
Bors E (1957) Neurogenic bladder. Urol Survey 7: 177–250
Bors E, Comarr E (1971) Neurologic urology, University Park Press, Baltimore
Bradley WE, Timm GW, Rockswold GL, Scott FB (1975) Detrusor and urethral electromyography.
    J Urol 114: 891–894
Coolsaet BLRA, Van Duyl WA, Van Mastrigt R, Van Der Swart A (1973) Stepwise cystometry.
    Urology 2: 255
Downie JW, Moochhala SM, Bialik JG (1983) The role of reflexes in modifying the response to
    bethanechol chloride. Neurourol Urodyn 2: 301
Giertz G, Lindbloom K (1951) Urethrocystographic studies of nervous disturbances of the urinary
    bladder and urethra. Acta Radiol 36: 205–216
Glahn BE (1970) Neurogenic bladder diagnosed pharmacologically on the basis of denervation
    supersensitivity. Scand Urol Nephrol 4: 13–15
Kiesswett H (1976) EMG-pattern of pelvic floor muscles with surface electrodes. Urol Int 31: 60–69
Klevmark B (1977) Motility of the urinary bladder in cats during filling at physiologic rates. Acta
    Physiol Scand 101: 176
Krane RJ Siroky MB (1979) Classification of neuro-urologic disorders In: Krane RJ, Siroky MB (eds)
    Clinical neuro-urology. Little Brown, Boston, pp 143–158
Lapides J (1976) Neuromuscular vesical and ureteral dysfunction. In: Campbell MF, Harrison JH (eds)
    Urology. Saunders Philadelphia
Lapides J, Friend CR, Ajemian EP, Reus WS (1962) Denervation supersensitivity as a test for
    neurogenic bladder. Surg Gynec Obstet 114: 241–244
Merrill DC, Rotta J (1983) A clinical evaluation of detrusor denervation supersensitivity using air
    cystometry. J Urol 111: 27–28
Muller LR (1902) Clinical and experimental studies of the innervation of the bladder. German J
    Neurology 21: 86–154
Munro D (1937) The treatment of the urinary bladder in cases with injury of the spinal cord. Am J
    Surg 38: 120–135
Nesbit RM, Baum WC (1954) Cystometry: its neurologic diagnostic implications. Neurology 4: 190–
    199
Nordling J, Meyhoff HH, Walter S, Andersen, JT (1978) Urethal electromyography using a new ring
    electrode. J Urol 120: 571
Pavlakis AJ, Siroky MB, Krane RJ (1983) Neurogenic detrusor areflexia: correlation of perineal elec-
    tromyography and bethanechol supersensitivity testing. J Urol 129: 1182–1183
Siroky MB, Krane RJ (1982) Neurologic aspects of detrusor sphincter dyssynergia with reference to
    the guarding reflex. J Urol 127: 953
Slater GS (1954) The neurogenic bladder. Postgrad Med 15: 18–23
Staskin D, Nehra A, Siroky M, Krane R (1988) Extended bladder pressure monitoring in spinal cord
    injured patient. Neurourol Urodyn 7: 191–192
Sundin T, Dahlstrom A, Norlen L et al. (1977) The sympathetic innervation and adrenoreceptor func-
    tion of the human lower urinary tract in the normal state and after parasympathetic denervation.
    Invest Urol 14: 322
Tang PC, Ruch TC (1955) Non-neurogenic basis of bladder tone. Am J Physiol 181: 249
Voris HC, Landes HE (1940) Cystometric studies in cases of neurologic disease. Arch Neurol Psychiatry
    44: 118–139
Wein AJ (1981) Classification of neurogenic voiding dysfunction. J Urol 125: 605
Wein AJ, Raezer DM, Malloy TR (1980) Failure of the bethanechol supersensitivity test to predict
    improved voiding after subcutaneous bethanechol administration. J Urol 123: 202
Yalla SV, Gittes RF (1977) Detrusor urethral sphincter dyssynergia. J Urol 118: 1026
Yalla SV, Rossier AB, Fam B (1976) Dysynergic vesicourethral responses during bladder rehabilita-
    tion in spinal cord injury patients. J Urol 115: 575

Difficulty with Voiding or Acute Urinary Retention Having Previously Voided Satisfactorily

K.F. Parsons

Introduction

Satisfactory micturition in spinal injured patients differs from that in the neurologically intact individual. The emphasis shifts from a physiological function which has to be socially acceptable in normal people, to that which is mandatory for preservation of the upper urinary tracts and avoidance of urinary infection, in patients with spinal injuries. This chapter addresses the problems encountered in patients in whom urethral voiding has been established following the initial management of their injury and yet present at a later stage with either acute urinary retention of with difficulty with micturition.

Identifying the Problem

There are three manifestations of voiding difficulties in spinal cord damaged patients. Urinary retention will be obvious; difficulty in micturition will be recognised and reported by the patient who will notice the problem directly or may identify an association of poor bladder emptying with autonomic dysreflexia and, finally, inefficient voiding may be detected by routine urological follow-up.

There is no doubt that the best assessors of whether the bladder is draining satisfactorily are often the patients themselves. Acute retention will be obvious, though clearly not manifest in the same painful way that afflicts the neurologically intact counterpart. Autonomic dysreflexia often heralds acute urinary retention and this diagnosis can readily be confirmed by a palpating hand on the abdomen. Thus diagnosed, rapid relief of retention is mandatory – see later.

Similarly, ineffective bladder emptying will often be suspected by the patient and this will be reported. It may be that the clue is a spurious odd sensation almost anywhere; an increase in peripheral spasm perhaps, or simply careful attention to the flow characteristics of voiding by the patient. Whatever the clues, it is as well for those who care for spinal injured patients to heed them.

In those cases where no such evidence is forthcoming, a safety net has to be planned to identify at an early stage any inadequacy of bladder emptying.

The first question to be answered for any spinal cord damaged patient is whether the method of bladder drainage remains satisfactory as time goes by. All patients should be on a carefully structured programme of urological follow-up to ensure that this is the case.

Just how this is achieved is perhaps controversial. The counsel of perfection is easy: all patient should have every possible urological test at each follow-up, as frequently and regularly as possible, to enable early detection of every potential problem. Common sense dictates that such an approach cannot be adopted. Thus a sensible programme must be initiated to use the most appropriate investigations to identify drainage problems, at intervals most likely to detect changes in bladder function before the whole urinary tract is compromised, with as minimum intervention and as little disruption as possible for the patient.

Screening Tests

Biochemical Assessment of Renal Function

Each patient should have an electrolyte assessment performed preferably every six months but at least at yearly intervals. However, only a serious deterioration in renal function will be highlighted by this method and indeed a single upper tract unit may be lost without any appreciable effect on overall renal function. Thus little reliance can be put on this test. It is perhaps surprising and gratifying how infrequently the upper urinary tracts are seriously compromised by bladder dysfunction in spinal injured patients provided that diligent attention is paid to regular follow-up of vesico-urethral function. (See Chapter 5.)

Urinary Tract Imaging

Intravenous Urography

The mainstay of urological follow-up in Spinal Injuries Units has been the intravenous urogram and there is no doubt that much information can be gleaned from serial urography in cord damaged patients (Chagnon et al. 1985). However, the cumulative radiation dose and the expense in time, both for the patient and the Spinal Unit, militate against this type of follow-up regimen.

Ultrasonography

Fortunately, the alternative method of assessment by ultrasonography is now available and in time may totally replace urography: Chagnon et al. (1985) found this method of investigation to be as reliable as intravenous urography in 92% of cases, and in 6% to supply additional information that was not apparent on urography. There are, inevitably, disadvantages with this imaging modality and they are these. The technique is totally "user dependent". This means that the ultrasonographer alone sees the best results of the technique, and "hard copy" of the pertinent results is difficult to obtain. The best glimpse of a thickened bladder wall may be difficult to freeze for a photograph of the scan to be taken. That being said, it may be argued that the medical staff of the Spinal Unit should acquire the expertise to perform the investigation and thus derive the maximum benefit from its use. Renal images are relatively easy to produce and will determine readily whether any upper tract dilatation is present and, similarly, residual bladder urine is easy to see. Bladder wall thickening is less obvious and may be of crucial importance in monitoring spinal injured cases, particularly those in whom outflow obstruction is developing to a significant degree.

Radionuclide Imaging

There is no doubt that renography with a radionuclide and gamma camera scanning will provide much information regarding renal parenchymal integrity and dynamic renal function. This, by inference, might forewarn when vesico-urethral dysfunction threatens the upper urinary tracts. It also can provide a crude assessment of post-voiding residual urine. The technique, however, is not readily available to Spinal Injuries Units, and often the difficulty in transferring patients with the disability which they have outweighs the benefit of such transfer to the Nuclear Medical Unit to use this imaging technique as a routine screening procedure. However, when dilatation of the upper urinary tract is found, isotope renography with diuresis certainly has a pivotal role in diagnosis and further management. (See Chapter 5.)

Direct Assessment of Bladder Function

The most accurate assessment available to determine efficacy of bladder function is directly to measure it by urodynamic assessment (Gardner et al. 1984). The most elementary of these investigations is direct measurement of the voided urinary flow rate. Unfortunately a simple uroflowmetric test is neither a technique which is practical to perform on spinal injured patients nor does it yield much useful information because the neuropathic bladder will not empty precisely to order as required in recording a uroflow-rate test.

Full urodynamic assessment, with or without synchronous radiographic screening, is therefore necessary and is described in detail in Chapter 3. Its disadvantage as a routine screening test is that it is an invasive investigation of considerable complexity but, as discussed below, it is mandatory in the diagnosis and selection of cases for treatment when vesico-urethral dysfunction is present.

Suggested Protocol of Monitoring

Upper Urinary Tract

Every spinal cord injured patient should be on a routine follow-up programme which includes a six-monthly assessment of renal function by biochemical analysis and yearly imaging study which assesses both the upper and lower urinary tracts. The imaging technique selected will vary depending upon the ease with which the investigation can be performed. Yearly follow-up by intravenous urography usually reveals early signs of potential compromise to an upper urinary tract unit before significant damage occurs. Yet experience at the Regional Spinal Injuries Centre at Southport has shown that, from a population of 850 patients on a regular follow-up programme using intravenous urography to monitor the upper tracts, three renal units have progressed from normality to non-function within a year as a result of midline bladder outflow obstruction. There is no particular correlation of this phenomenon with the neurological level nor, interestingly, is a long interval after injury a protector against it. It has been observed in a patient in a neurologically and apparently urologically stable state for some eight years after injury. Early detection of this pathological process is of the utmost importance and perhaps frequent, regular ultrasound screening will provide the answer when the merest hint of dilatation in a previously normal upper tract should be pursued as vigorously as possible. (See Chapter 5.)

Lower Urinary Tract

Screening programmes to detect lower urinary tract dysfunction should include a regular assessment of the residual urine and if possible of bladder wall thickness. Ultrasound examination is ideal for the former but the latter is rather harder to detect by this method. It can be inferred by scrunity of a plain abdominal X-ray when, if a bladder "shadow" can be seen, the inference is that thickening of the detrusor is responsible for the radiodensity (Timoney et al. 1989). From the area of the shadow an approximation of the residual urine can be calculated. Diligent attempts at emptying the bladder should always be made therefore, before a plain radiograph is taken, if this radiological sign is to be of value.

A specific and detailed analysis of voiding efficiency can be made by a comprehensive urodynamic investigation (Chapter 3). A full pressure-flow urodynamic study on spinal cord injured patients requires considerable patience and skill but when properly performed will produce the most accurate data regarding vesico-urethral function.

Urethral Pressure Profilometry

This urostatic investigation potentially can identify external sphincter/intrinsic urethral dyssynergia and by using pharmacological blocking agents differentiate between the two (Sham Sunder et al. 1978; Thomas et al. 1984).

Dynamic Voiding Pressure Profilometry.   This extends the technique to allow precise identification of the level of midline outflow obstruction. The technique involves plotting a urethral profile *during* micturition, and analysing the pressure separation measured by a second transducer within the bladder which monitors intravesical pressure continuously. The separation occurs because of the drop in pressure which takes place across the site of obstruction within the outflow tract. This point of separation can readily be correlated with cursors set on a static urethral pressure profile curve so that the anatomical level of obstruction can be identified with confidence (Desmond and Ramayya 1988). Of those patients with spinal injuries, the technique is limited to paraplegic patients, because movement artefacts invalidate the data and thus preclude tetraplegics who have a propensity to spasm. It holds the great advantage that it will identify the level of outflow obstruction without recourse to radiological screening.

Treatment Options

Acute Urinary Retention

The management of the bladder in a patient who develops acute retention of urine having previously been voiding satisfactorily is, of course, identical to that which is invoked at the time of acute spinal injury. Decompression is an acute emergency and should be undertaken as quickly as possible. The options are threefold. Catheterisation may be per urethram and indwelling; per urethram and intermittent; or suprapubic. Each will have their advocates and there are valid reasons for selecting a particular method and each will be considered briefly.

Indwelling Urethral Catheterisation

This remains the mainstay of treatment of retention in both males and females. Fine-diameter catheters should always be used, with a high ratio of internal to external diameter. Thought must be given to the time for which the catheter is likely to be left in place and, if it is to be prolonged, silicone catheters should be used. Unfortunately these catheters do not have a particularly large internal diameter, but the diminished reaction which they provoke within the urethra when compared to latex catheters provides a great advantage. It is as well to remember that *silicone-coated* latex catheters manufactured in an attempt to match the properties of pure silicone catheters lose the coating within 24 hours within the urethra, thus negating any advantage which silicone coating may have (Blacklock 1986).

The weight of the tubing and drainage bag must always be supported, especially in females. If attention is not paid to this simple detail, damage by pressure necrosis at the bladder neck in females progressing ultimately to complete destruction of the whole of the urethra will occur. In males, if the catheter and tubing are not supported, a "bow-string" of the urethra will occur producing a urethral stricture at the site of maximum pressure against the urethral wall.

It must be accepted that the intravesical foreign body of a indwelling catheter will provoke lower urinary tract infection if present for more than three days or so, but antibacterial therapy should be withheld unless systemic effects of infection become manifest.

Intermittent Catheterisation

With the realisation that urinary infection was rendered less likely when the bladder was drained regularly and completely came the re-institution of the technique of intermittent catheterisation for patients with inefficient bladder emptying (Lapides et al. 1972). This method of bladder drainage can be used in spinal cord injured patients with acute retention, but involves organisational problems which are especially troublesome in tetraplegic patients who are unable to catheterise themselves. The technique, though simple in concept, has to be carefully taught and practised with great diligence. Once adopted there can be no respite, for the bladder must be emptied at regular four-hourly intervals during the waking hours. Nonetheless this method of bladder drainage has revolutionised the management of the neuropathic bladder.

Suprapubic Catheterisation

Suprapubic catheterisation is an attractive logical answer to the problem of retention and will leave the urethra uninstrumented and theoretically uncontaminated. It requires skill to perform and carries with it a certain morbidity. The colon and peritoneum are both vulnerable, yet serious damage is fortunately a rarity. Theoretically at least, suprapubic tracks may re-open if, once voiding is re-established, the bladder develops outflow obstruction as it potentially may do in spinal injured patients.

Subsequent Management

As soon as the bladder is drained satisfactorily, attention must be focused on the cause of retention. It is a truism that greater numbers of spinal injured male patients are surviving to the age where benign prostatic hyperplasia may develop and this of course is a possible aetiology of urinary retention in a patient who previously was voiding satisfactorily. Interestingly, however, the prostate gland does not seem to grow to any great extent in patients with vesico-urethral neuropathy though the reason why it should not do so is not clear.

The probability is, therefore, that retention or voiding difficulty is due to minor or marginal changes in the balance between the forces of expulsion and those of continence, the neurological control of which is decentralised by the spinal injury. Neurological progression is certainly a possibility but beyond the first three months of injury (dealt with in Chapter 2) the neurological status has usually stabilised. Nonetheless a full neurological assessment is mandatory and any neurological change detected.

In the absence of a change in the neurological status of the patient, a search for other causes of retention should be made. These include urinary tract infection, which although never a cause of retention in neurologically intact patients can provoke retention in spinal injured patients perhaps due to the inhibitory effect on smooth muscle by bacterial toxins.

Constipation is both a potent cause of retention and is common, if not universal, in spinal injured patients and thus should be specifically excluded or, when present, be corrected before the vesico-urethral apparatus is investigated in detail. Finally, acute peri-anal conditions such as an anal fissure may provoke retention and must thus also be excluded.

The basic concept of "a trial of micturition" is appropriate in these patients and this should be undertaken once any precipitating factor causing retention has been corrected. Clearly, it is vital that an objective assessment of the adequacy of bladder emptying in this "trial" circumstance is made. The examining hand is insufficient and a careful check on post-micturitional residual urine volumes must be made, preferably after several voids over a period of days. This may best be performed by ultrasound examination, but it is also justified to check the residual by catheter, so important is it to be certain that a satisfactory micturition pattern has been established before the patient is discharged home.

Surgical Intervention

If the situation arises that a satisfactory micturition pattern is not achieved, then intervention will have to be contemplated (Fig. 4.1). The mainstay in determining the management of the neuropathic bladder must be the results of a full urodynamic assessment of vesico-urethral activity. (See Chapter 3.)

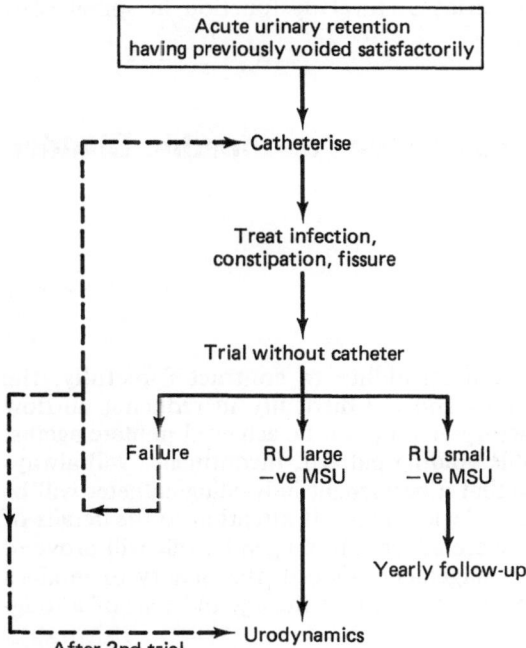

Figure 4.1 Algorithm indicating management of acute retention. (From Gardner BP, Parsons KF, Machin DG, Galloway A, Krishnan KR (1986) Urological management of spinal cord damaged patients. Paraplegia 24: 138–147.)

The urodynamic patterns which determine treatment can pragmatically be categorised into relatively simple groups. The fundamental phenomena are three: whether the detrusor exhibits any contractility; whether that contractility satisfactorily opens the bladder neck; and whether urethral resistance to flow, be that by intermittent disco-ordinated pelvic floor contractions or by similar unwanted intrinsic urethral muscular contraction, exceeds the contractile force of the detrusor.

In lower motor neurone lesions the "expulsive force" is provided by abdominal straining and the inappropriate urethral resistance results from contraction of intrinsic urethral muscle, whereas in higher lesions the detrusor will usually, if not always, regain uninhibited contractility whilst urethral resistance is a combination of disco-ordinated striated and intrinsic muscular activity.

Therefore, the *neuropathic urethra* is the critical element which has to be treated in vesico-urethral neuropathy. If the expulsive force is sufficient, the resistance in the urethra is the crucial and fundamental factor (Gibbon et al. 1980). There are differences in the treatment of abnormal micturition in spinal cord injured patients depending upon the type of neuropathic vesico-urethral dysfunction exhibited and, inevitably, differences in the treatment of males and females.

The activity of the autonomic muscle of the urinary tract can readily be modified by drug therapy and this provides a treatment option which may be considered. Authoritative reviews are available and another publication in this series, *Pharmacological Management of the Urinary Tract*, edited by Marco Caine, is devoted to the topic. Further detailed consideration of drug therapy as primary treatment for neuropathic vesico-urethral dysfunction in spinal cord injuries will thus not be undertaken.

Surgical Management of the Female Neuropathic Bladder

Suprasacral Lesions

Catheterisation

Even though the detrusor may retain an ability to contract forcefully, the uninhibited nature of the contractions and the difficulty in reducing outflow resistance to the point where satisfactory voiding can be achieved militate against successful restoration of a reasonable voiding pattern. Incontinence will always occur and it is most likely therefore that a permanent indwelling catheter will be the best treatment option for the tetraplegic female. If attention to the details of catheter management indicated above are adhered to diligently, this will prove to be the most satisfactory form of management. Indeed, the quality of modern catheters and of catheter management are such that the age-old fear of a long-term catheter has evaporated.

If, when catheterised, the bladder exhibits excessive contractility to produce bypassing, then treatment to inhibit detrusor activity is required. Antimuscarinic anticholinergic agents are indicated. Oxybutinin hydrochloride is perhaps the most effective but is available on a "named patient" basis only in the United Kingdom.

Terodiline – an anticholinergic calcium channel antagonist – is more readily available.

Peripheral mass somatic spasms will often also provoke bypass leakage and thus drug therapy with skeletal muscle relaxants with baclofen, a centrally acting benzodiazepine, or dantrolene, which acts directly on striated muscle, will be beneficial.

Surgical Intervention

Surgical procedures to inhibit detrusor contractility might be considered. Ablation of the vesical pelvic nerves by transtrigonal phenol injection seems less effective in tetraplegic spinal injured patients than it does in patients suffering with demyelinating diseases (Ewing et al. 1983). Transvaginal neurotomy similarly has not proved adequate to control neuropathic hyperreflexia and bladder transection also is inadequate. A more aggressive pudendal neurectomy, sacral rhizotomy, intrathecal phenol or conectomy might be appropriate and should be considered where the hyperreflexic bladder activity proves to be particularly disabling, particularly when associated with peripheral somatic spasms.

An attractive option in female patients with suprasacral neuropathic bladder dysfunction might be to perform a cutaneous urinary diversion with an ileal conduit. The obvious disadvantage is that the patient is quite unable to manage the stoma appliance without help because of upper limb paralysis. Furthermore, the long-term results of simple diversion in other groups are proving to be disappointing and thus with hindsight it transpires that not to have used this operation was, and remains, entirely justified, particularly as life expectancy in spinal cord injured patients is increasing.

Sacral Lesions

The configuration of the filling cystometrogram in patients with a sacral neuropathic bladder is of fundamental importance. If compliance is low, and it may be so due to a mechanism which is incompletely understood, it is essential to choose a method of bladder drainage which does not allow the intrinsic bladder pressure to exceed 45 cmH$_2$O for any prolonged period. Failure to observe this criterion will produce damage to the upper urinary tracts (see Chapters 3 and 5). To increase compliance, drug therapy with anticholinergic agents may be necessary and has been shown to be effective (Thompson and Lauvetz 1976). Alternatively, a bowel interpositional cystoplasty to increase capacity and compliance may be contemplated. In the author's experience, however, this operation has never been necessary in spinal cord injured patients, in direct contradistinction to patients with congenital lesions of the lumbo-sacral spine. This perhaps is a reflection that the growing decentralised bladder exhibits different visco-elastic characteristics than does a normal bladder deprived acutely of its innervation.

Clean Intermittent Catheterisation

The optimum management for the majority of female patients with a sacral neuropathic bladder is to use a regimen of clean intermittent catheterisation. This method of bladder drainage was universal in the late 1930s and early 1940s for patients whose bladders were rendered neuropathic by an abdomino-perineal excision of the rectum (Lockhart-Mummery and Norbury 1932). It fell into disrepute, however, because of the extraordinary high incidence of sepsis which was produced. Guttman and Frankel (1966) instituted a regimen of intermittent catheterisation in spinal cord injured patients, with strict attention to sterility at every catheterisation. Lapides, however, popularised the technique of "clean" intermittent self catheterisation in the early 1960s for the management of the acontractile neuropathic bladder in children. The logic of the technique came with the realisation that bacterial infection of the intermittently catheterised bladder did not ensue provided that it was emptied completely on a regular basis. Any bacteria within the bladder were eliminated and would thus not have the opportunity to divide and thrive (Lapides et al. 1972).

This simple prerequisite that *regular* intermittent catheterisation should replace *normal* voiding permitted the use of a socially *clean* catheter rather than the notion that previously had been held that any instrumentation of the urethra for whatever purpose should be instruments or catheters which were surgically sterile.

Urethral Overdilatation

There is, however, the potential for preservation of urethral voiding in females with sacral neuropathic bladder dysfunction and this option should always be remembered for those patients who cannot or will not intermittently catheterise themselves. Abdominal straining may provide an expulsive force sufficient to open the bladder neck and urethra and to allow emptying. Some form of reduction of excessive urethral resistance may be required. In these cases, intrinsic urethral contractility is the culprit, for there is no striated muscle activity by the very nature of the neural lesion. Indeed, it is because the pelvic floor is flaccid that abdominal pressure is detracted from the urethra as the pelvic floor "blows out" that allows the urethra to open. Reduction in urethral resistance may be achieved pharmacologically with alpha-adrenoreceptor blockade or by urethral overdistension. The latter physically disrupts the integrity of the intrinsic spiral muscle fibres within the urethra and thus reduces the resistance which they impart. If this form of treatment is chosen it must be remembered that the diameter to which the urethra should be stretched is large and should be at least to a size which will easily accept the little finger within the urethral lumen. This type of overdilatation is best achieved with Hawkins-Ambler dilators for they have a gradual increase in diameter from the rounded tip to the shoulder of the instrument at its maximum diameter which facilitates urethral overstretching. If the urethra is not dilated to such a large diameter, the procedure will be ineffective.

If the bladder neck is competent, urethral overdilatation will not provoke stress-induced incontinence. Paradoxically, the procedure may cure stress-induced leakage from a chronically overdistended bladder in which the bladder neck is constantly pulled open by the excessive volume by allowing complete emptying by abdominal straining.

Other Options

It is tempting to suppose that resection of the bladder neck in females with sacral vesico-urethral neuropathy will facilitate voiding by straining, particularly as the level of obstruction seems to declare itself on video-urodynamics at the bladder neck. Indeed, bladder neck resection has been used in the past in just this circumstance with some success but the risk of incontinence is so great that this operation is best avoided in females, particularly as the option of clean intermittent catheterisation is infinitely preferable.

Restoration of Bladder Neck Competence

Loss of support of the pelvic floor which will allow transmitted abdominal pressure to be deflected away from the urethra (see above) may in time render the bladder neck incompetent and stress-induced urinary leakage will ensue. Some form of surgical restoration of the bladder neck and proximal urethra back under the compressive influence of abdominal pressure will be required. A simple "Stamey" needle suspension of the vagina either side of the bladder neck might suffice though in extreme cases an open suprapubic colposuspension operation is required. Surgery such as this should only be undertaken in those cases in whom intermittent catheterisation can readily be used for it will invariably be necessary at least in the early postoperative period if not permanently.

Surgical Management of the Male Neuropathic Bladder

Suprasacral Lesions

The bladder which is totally decentralised at a spinal level well above the sacral micturition centre will regain contractility in an uninhibited hyperreflexic fashion. This will be either with normal compliance during progressive filling or with reduced compliance producing an inexorable pressure rise as the bladder fills. In addition, uninhibited pressures waves may be exhibited. Urine is only retained within the bladder if the midline outflow resistance exceeds the intravesical pressure. This midline resistance is exerted at either the level of the bladder neck, at the level of the membranous urethra, or both. The forces which produce the pressure resistance at the level of the membranous urethra comprise either: intrinsic urethral muscle contractility; dyssynergic striated pelvic floor muscle activity; or a combination of both.

Urodynamic studies which include videocystography are crucial in determining the level and extent of midline outflow obstruction (Chapter 3) and are thus mandatory in selecting treatment options (Fig. 4.2).

There is a fundamental decision to be made at the outset of determining treatment for a male (usually young) with suprasacral neuropathic vesico-urethral dysfunction. The options are whether to leave the midline vesico-urethral apparatus untouched and artificially to stimulate voiding using a sacral anterior root stimulator (Brindley et al. 1986), or whether to reduce or ablate the midline resistance and produce unobstructed, uninhibited voiding per urethram to be collected in a condom urinal device.

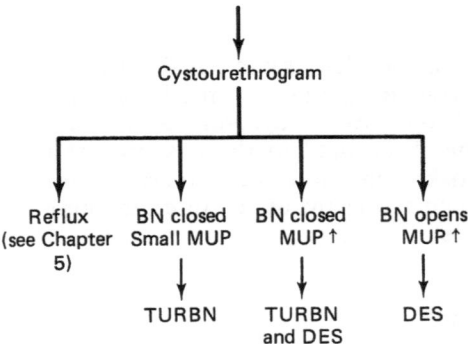

Figure 4.2 Algorithm indicating surgical options in midline outflow obstruction. BN, bladder neck; MUP, maximal urethral pressure; TURBN, transurethral resection of bladder neck; DES, division of external urethral sphincter. (From Gardner BP, Parsons KF, Machin DG, Galloway A, Krishnan KR (1986) Paraplegia 24: 138–147.)

The use of sacral anterior root stimulators is discussed extensively in Chapter 9 and will not be considered further.

The endoscopic surgical treatment options briefly are threefold: incision or resection of the bladder neck; incision of the distal urethral mechanism (external sphincterotomy); or both.

Bladder Neck Resection

The prostate gland does not seem to undergo hyperplasia in spinal injured man with the same frequency as his neurologically intact counterpart, and therefore, if bladder neck obstruction is diagnosed, it is resection of just the bladder neck which is usually required. However, the operation should only be contemplated by surgeons well practised in endoscopic surgical techniques and who are able readily to remove the whole prostate gland endoscopically if required. All the usual prerequisites of this type of surgery are mandatory. Antibacterial prophylaxis should always be used whether or not preoperative urine cultures are positive because patients with vesico-urethral neuropathy who have had any type of instrumentation whatever at any stage seem always to have a significantly higher tendency to bacteraemia, endotoxaemia or septicaemia following endoscopic surgery.

When bladder neck obstruction is diagnosed surgical correction can be either by incision or resection. Bladder neck incision, however, does not seem totally to relieve obstruction in these cases, and a formal resection is always preferable. A circumferential resection is unnecessary and in any event will increase the incidence of postoperative bladder neck sclerosis. An anterior mucosal bridge should therefore always be retained to prevent this tedious complication of bladder neck resection. This principle matches that of mucosal preservation at haemorrhoidectomy which has the similar benefit of prevention of anal cicatrisation following that operation.

The resection should always be deep, leaving only a thin rim of circumferentially orientated bladder neck fibres. It is preferable to avoid resecting into the extravesical fat at this level, and to avoid undermining the trigone, but care must be taken to excavate posterior fibres as thinly as possible or a shelf of tissue will be retained which will make postoperative catheterisation, if ever required, very much more difficult.

If hyperplasia of the prostate gland is present, the adenomata should be excavated to the level of the capsule at all areas. The simplest way of assessing the adequacy of such a resection is to examine the residual prostatic capsule by rectal palpation, where it should be felt as no more than the merest capsular rim. If any hyperplastic prostatic tissue is felt, even after observing what appears endoscopically to be a complete resection, further resection is mandatory until all the adenoma is completely removed (Gibbon 1978). This does not usually sacrifice the anterior mucosal strip for adenomatous growth does not extend in the midline anteriorly in the smaller gland. Complete excavation of the gland has the added benefit of allowing the capsular fibres to contract once all the adenomatous tissue has been removed so that a natural haemostatic mechanism is brought into play. This may be augmented by pressure on the capsule by an intrarectal finger which will produce almost immediate cessation of any venous bleeding (Freyer 1901; Gibbon 1978) which sometimes proves difficult to control by coagulation diathermy. Finally, diligent removal of all intraurethral adenoma militates against regrowth of the gland.

Postoperative catheterisation with irrigation either by a three-way catheter, or by augmented diuresis, should always be used because it is vital that blockage should never occur for this will induce profound autonomic dysreflexia with the potential risk that any hypertension thus provoked might initiate further haemorrhage from the prostatic bed.

The catheter should be retained in place for a day or two longer than normally is required for a neurologically intact patient undergoing prostatectomy, even if the irrigant or urine is crystal clear, for the vagaries of bladder function are such that once a trial of micturition is commenced, there will be more frequent and vigorous contraction of the prostatic capsule and thus a potential tendency to further bleeding is present. This can be lessened if a mature eschar, or even early re-epithelialisation of the raw bladder neck and prostatic area, is well under way.

On removal of the catheter, the output from the bladder must be monitored closely, and the residual urine checked, preferably by ultrasound examination. If a satisfactory pattern is not quickly established, the catheter must be replaced for a day or two more.

Incision of the Distal Urethral Mechanism – External Sphincterotomy

If the external sphincter region is compromised in any way during endoscopic prostatic surgery in a neurologically intact man, dribbling incontinence with the bladder permanently empty is the inevitable outcome. Yet to achieve just such a state of incontinence and to overcome urethral outflow resistance by ablation of the sphincteric mechanism in neuropathic cases can be extraordinarily difficult – one of the strange perversities of urological surgery.

The operation of external sphincterotomy, perhaps more properly defined as internal membranous urethrotomy, is designed to abolish neuropathic urethral outflow obstruction. This applies whether that obstruction is due to spasticity and overactivity of the striated pelvic floor or whether the obstructing element is due solely to increased activity in the intrinsic urethral muscle. Indeed the first cases of "external sphincterotomy" reported by Ross and Gibbon were performed for urethral obstruction in patients with flaccid paraparesis (Ross et al. 1957). The precise cause of the obstruction had not been determined; the theory initially was that a concertina effect in the region of the membranous urethra was responsible, producing the so-called "curtsey sign" (Vincent 1966). Be that as it may, sphincterotomy was successful and voiding facilitated in these cases. Subsequent work has shown the obstruction to be in the intrinsic urethral muscle itself, which appears to have an alpha-adrenoreceptor nerve supply and which demonstrates a denervation or decentralisation supersensitivity (Parsons and Turton 1980; Gibbon et al. 1980).

Having determined that "sacral" neuropathic urethral obstruction could be satisfactorily abolished by external sphincterotomy the procedure was later applied to "suprasacral" lesions where the obstruction was rather more evidently due to abnormal muscular contraction of the periurethral somatic and intrinsic urethral muscle.

Operative Technique

The operation is the same whatever the cause of the obstruction. The choice of anaesthesia will depend on the case to be operated upon (see Chapter 8). A relaxed lithotomy position should always be used and antibacterial prophylaxis always given (see above).

Whether an irrigating or a standard resectoscope is used is left to the surgeon's preference though if an irrigating system is selected it is mandatory to reduce the suction of the outflow to a minimum, for the perisphincteric mucosa will otherwise be sucked into the outflow ports during endourethral manipulation. The resulting ischaemia, albeit temporary, will increase the chance of a secondary stricture at this level.

It must be decided at which points the incisions in the sphincteric apparatus are to be made. The options are to divide by a single incision posterolaterally; by posterobilateral incisions; or to use a single incision of the sphincter in the midline at the 12 o'clock position. Consideration of each option should be given. A single posterolateral sphincteric incision does not ablate sphincteric activity as efficiently as does this type of incision at the bladder neck. The explanation is perhaps that the fibres do not spring apart and that restorative healing allows reactivation of sphincteric action. A posterobilateral incision is thus preferable. This will ensure as far as possible that the divided sphincter will not reobstruct. The disadvantage of this operation is that the incision through the urethral muscle occurs at precisely the point at which the nerves to the corpora cavernosa traverse the membranous region (Walsh and Donker 1982). Postoperative erectile failure is thus a much more likely complication. Published studies have failed to demonstrate such an outcome but nonetheless the author prefers to avoid this type of sphincterotomy if there is any question of preservation of erectile function. A midline sphincterotomy is thus used in such cases.

The surgery is relatively simple. It is vital that endoscopic landmarks are determined with accuracy and confidence and that the operator has sufficient experience never to lose those landmarks even if haemorrhage ensues. The verumontanum is the anatomical key to the procedure. All muscle layers in the urethra must be divided from a level a little above the veru to some 2 to 2.5 cm below it. These distances are purely arbitrary and with experience the operator will know precisely to which point the muscle incision must extend. It is a little easier to define the sphincter when the posterolateral incisions are chosen, for a median sphincterotomy requires an anterior incision in the convex curve of the urethra through and below the sphincter which is more difficult to visualise accurately.

The cut must be made through all muscle layers and some authors advise that it be made with a "Collins" or "bee sting" electrode using the coagulation current (Gibbon 1982). This unfortunately will char the tissue and tend to make it adhere to the electrode which hinders the procedure. If the cutting current is used, a crisp incision can be made but care must be taken not to cut too aggressively for the corpus spongiosum will be opened deeply and will bleed furiously. Some degree of spongiosal bleeding is frequently encountered and cannot be stopped by coagulation even with a large roller ball electrode. In this circumstance it will invariably stop by tamponade using a large-diameter catheter, so a 24 F catheter is justified in these cases. Traction on the retaining balloon is quite unnecessary. The author's preference is to use a catheter without a retaining balloon and to fix it with retaining external straps – the Gibbon catheter. If postoperative bleeding fails to cease promptly, a combination of a rectal finger compression and pressure in the perineum will guarantee haemostasis. Postoperative irrigation should always be used for it is imperative that the catheter does not block and that dysreflexia is avoided.

An indwelling catheter should be retained for at least five or six days and upon removal the strictest attention paid to the adequacy of voiding.

Sphincterotomy Failure

There is no doubt that in a small number of cases external sphincterotomy fails to achieve satisfactory bladder emptying. The precise cause of this failure is not well understood, and it is tempting to assume that fibrosis and scarring of the urethral muscle are responsible. There is, however, some evidence that the intrinsic urethral muscle regains an ability to contract and that alpha-adrenoreceptor blockade will abolish the sphincteric peak observed in sphincterotomy failure cases (Ross et al. 1976). There is no reason why the procedure should not be repeated, but little doubt that fibrosis will ultimately ensue if several attempts at endoscopic sphincterotomy are made.

Other Options

The goal of endoscopic surgery on the external urethral sphincter is to reduce totally the resistance which it imparts to urethral flow of urine. The same objective can be achieved by *stenting* the sphincter in an open attitude. This approach is in its very infancy but it would appear that the insertion of a urethral wall stent (A.M.S. Medical, UK Ltd.) holds the sphincter open and has produced satisfactory results (McInerney et al. 1990), though as yet its use has been confined to those cases in which external sphincterotomy has failed. Long-term assessment of this type of treatment is awaited.

The surgical procedures detailed in this chapter should be used within the constraints of the fundamental principle which dominates the philosophy of management of the urinary tract in spinal cord damaged patients in that *preservation of renal function is always paramount*.

References

Blacklock NJ (1986) Catheters and urethral strictures. Br J Urol 58: 475–478

Brindley GS, Polkey CE, Rushton DN Cardozo L (1986) Sacral anterior root stimulation for bladder control in paraplegics – the first 50 cases. J Neurol Neurosurg Psychiatry 49: 1104–1114

Chagnon S, Vallee C, Laissy JP, Blery M (1985) Comparison of ultrasound and intravenous urography imaging of the urinary tract for investigation of 50 patients with spinal cord injuries. J Radiol 66(12): 801–806

Desmond AD, Ramayya GR (1988) Comparison of pressure flow studies with micturitional urethral pressure profiles in the diagnosis of urinary outflow obstruction. Br J Urol 61: 224–229

Ewing R, Bultitude MI, Shuttleworth KED (1983) Subtrigonal phenol injection therapy for incontinence in female patients with multiple sclerosis. Lancet 1: 1304–1305

Freyer PJ (1901) Total extirpation of the prostate for radical cure of enlargement of that gland. Br Med J 2: 125–129

Gardner BP, Parsons KF, Machin DG, Jameson RM, Krishnan KR (1984) The role of urodynamics in the management of spinal cord injured patients. Paraplegia 22: 157–161

Gibbon NOK (1978) Prostatectomy. In Hadfield J, Hobsley M (eds) Current surgical practice vol 2. Edward Arnold, Hodder & Stoughton, London, pp 283–298

Gibbon NOK (1982) Operative management of vesicourethral neuropathy. In: Rob and Smith's Operative urology. Butterworths, London, pp 406–409

Gibbon NOK, Parsons KF, Woolfenden KA (1980) The neuropathic urethra. Paraplegia 18: 221–225

Guttman L, Frankel H (1966) The value of intermittent catheterisation in the early management of traumatic paraplegia and tetraplegia. Paraplegia 4: 63–84

Lapides J, Diokno AC, Silber SJ, Lowe BS (1972) Clean, intermittent self catheterisation in the treatment of urinary tract disease. J Urol 107: 458–461

Lockhart-Mummery JP, Norbury LEC (1932) Discussion on urinary complications of diseases of the large intestine. Proc R Soc Med 8(1): 1820–1833

McInerney PD, Powell CS, Vanner TF, Stephenson TP (1990) Permanent urethral stents for detrusor sphincter dyssynergia. Presented at the 46th meeting Br Assoc Urol Surg, Scarborough (abstr)

Parsons KF, Turton M (1980) Urethral supersensitivity and occult urethral neuropathy. Br J Urol 52: 200–203

Ross JC, Gibbon NOK, Damanski M (1957) Resection of the external sphincter in the paraplegic – a preliminary report. Trans Am Assoc Genitourin Surg 69: 193–198

Ross JC, Gibbon NOK, Sham Sunder G (1976) Division of the external urethral sphincter in the neuropathic bladder – a twenty years review Br J Urol 48: 649–656

Sham Sunder G, Parsons KF, Gibbon NOK (1978) Outflow obstruction in neuropathic bladder dysfunction: the neuropathic urethra. Br J Urol 50: 190–199

Stott MA (1990) Compliance in the neuropathic bladder. MD Thesis, the University of Bristol

Thomas DG, Philip NH, McDermott TE, Rickwood AM (1984) The use of urodynamic studies to assess the effect of pharmacological agents with particular reference to alpha-adrenergic blockade. Paraplegia 22: 162–167

Thompson IM, Lauvetz R (1976) Oxybutinin in bladder spasm, neurogenic bladder and enuresis. Urology 8 (5): 452–454

Timoney, AG, Payne SR, Davies LAL, Abercrombie GF (1989) The plain film bladder shadow in outflow obstruction: as accurate a discriminant of residual urine as ultrasound. Br J Urol 63: 363–366

Vincent SA (1966) Some aspects of bladder mechanics. Biomed Eng, Sept 1–8

Walsh PC, Donker PJ (1982) Impotence following radical prostatectomy: insight into etiology and prevention. J Urol 128: 492–497

Chapter 5

Upper Urinary Tract Dilatation and Stones

B.P. Gardner and K.F. Parsons

Introduction

There has been a profound change in the survival of patients with spinal injuries since the advent of specialised units dedicated to the care of these unfortunate patients. Soon after the first world war, it became evident that renal failure as a result of upper urinary tract obstruction and/or urosepsis was the prime cause of mortality. The gratifying change in the mortality has been carefully recorded over the last 30 years. In 1961 it was found to be around 50% (Breithaupt et al. 1961). By 1968 the mortality figure had dropped to 36% (Jousse et al. 1968) and yet a further drop was found in 1973 at 30.8% (Geisler et al. 1977). Renal failure was still at this point the leading cause of death, and the death rate from it approximately three times that of the normal population.

The marked decrease in renal deaths continued when in 1983 it stood at 15.3% (Geisler et al. 1983). Of course the concurrent advent of renal replacement therapy which is available to spinal cord injured patients will have had a significant effect on mortality figures, but nonetheless careful urological management has had a substantial impact to the point where in the nineties, renal compromise is a rarity, possibly no more prevalent than 1% of cases and certainly not the common cause of death that it formerly was.

Upper Tract Dilatation

The essence of prevention of upper tract complications lies in the monitoring programme. The upper tracts can be followed morphologically, or functionally.

Morphological Monitoring

In Chapter 4 the relative merits of morphological follow-up by intravenous urography or by ultrasonography are discussed. Using a programme of ultrasonographic follow-up it has been possible at the Spinal Injuries centre, Southport to monitor 20% of all tetraplegics, in the community. A hidden advantage of this policy is that the defaulting rate is much lower. In general, on the previous programme which relied solely upon regular intravenous urography, there was a 25% non-attendance rate among 850 patients on the programme, largely and indeed fortunately, because of the patients' well being.

Whichever modality is chosen, it is mandatory that some assessment of the upper tracts is made at least yearly. Perhaps with ultrasonographic examinations, assessment may be made more frequently.

The aim of any morphological examination is to detect early signs of dilatation either unilaterally or bilaterally so that corrective treatment can be prompt. This of course raises a criticism of ultrasonography which is unable to detect ureteric dilatation until it is particularly gross and thus will be less sensitive than intravenous urography in this circumstance.

Functional Monitoring

There are two methods of functional upper tract assessment. The first, which is relatively crude, is to monitor overall renal function by biochemical analysis. Perhaps 90% of overall renal function must be lost before there will be any alteration in either urea or creatinine, and of course a unilateral upper tract can be lost entirely without any alteration in these parameters. It must therefore be recognised that little reliance should be placed on biochemical assessment in isolation but it should be used in conjunction with morphological studies.

Direct measurement of upper tract function can be made by radionuclide studies with gamma camera renography (O'Reilly et al. 1986). Undoubtedly this investigation is the most helpful in estimating the degree of renal damage and the potential for recovery. However, there are substantial difficulties in performing this test on spinal injured patients. They include those of access to the Nuclear Medical Unit by the patient and, because of deformity, to the patient by the gamma camera. Finally, clarity of an image collected over a period of several minutes in a patient who inadvertently may move as a result of mass somatic spasm may be less than optimum. Despite these disadvantages, the investigation is essential in both difficult and in subtle cases of upper tract obstruction, and perhaps rather more importantly in determining when the dilated upper tract is *not* obstructed but merely hypercompliant. To diagnose this circumstance with confidence the technique of "diuresis renography" (O'Reilly et al. 1986) should be used.

Causes of Upper Tract Dilatation

Upper urinary tract dilatation in spinal cord injured patients is usually asymptomatic and discovered by routine urological follow-up. There are a variety of causes:

Chronic Bacterial Infection. Perhaps by paralysing the urinary tract smooth muscle by endotoxins, chronic bacterial infection may be responsible and it is thus of the utmost importance that these patients have regular bacteriological surveillance. (See Chapter 6.) Isotope renography will determine that there is no obstructive lesion present when the radionuclide will be cleared after a diuretic challenge. This situation of upper tract dilatation without obstruction is an uncommon finding in spinal cord damaged patients.

Vesico-ureteric Reflux. This may be transient or permanent and therefore more sinister. It becomes commoner the longer after the spinal injury, and is found in a higher proportion of suprasacral lesions than sacral lesions with an overall incidence as high as 17% (Cosbie Ross 1965). It has been speculated that preservation of the sympathetic outflow to the trigone in these latter cases may have a protective effect upon trigonal function and thus allow the ureteric orifices to maintain their valvular function (Bors 1954), though the interruption of the parasympathetic outflow to the bladder and pelvic floor seems to exhibit a protective effect perhaps because abdominal straining to void will enhance intramural ureteric closure.

In spinal cord damaged patients, just as in neurologically intact children, urinary tract infection can produce reflux, be perseverated by it, and when eliminated cause the reflux to cease. Infected urine in a refluxing system is a potent cause of fever in spinal cord injured patients and a high index of suspicion must therefore be maintained and appropriate cystography performed to make the diagnosis in those cases where videocystography is not part of routine urodynamic evaluation.

Intramural Ureteric Obstruction. This may occur as the ureter passes through a thickened bladder wall. The ureter may be especially vulnerable at this site when fibrosis of the bladder wall is present. Invariably these cases are associated with midline outflow obstruction and thus the diagnosis should be suspected when upper tract dilatation does not resolve after outflow surgery. Scarring of the mucosal orifice itself, as a result of chronic infection, is a further cause of this category of obstruction.

Midline Bladder Outflow Obstruction. This is by far the commonest cause of upper tract dilatation in neuropathic cases. There is evidence that if the intravesical pressure is allowed to remain above 45 cmH$_2$O for any sustained periods then upper tract dilatation will ensue. Recent studies have suggested that low compliance alone is not necessarily the predetermining factor and that the configuration of the filling cystometrogram may predict upper tract dilatation. Those cases in which uninhibited pressure waves during filling are demonstrated carry with them the highest risk of upper tract dilatation in a manner similar to cases of chronic urinary retention in neurologically intact patients (Machin et al. 1985).

Stones. These may obstruct the ureter and produce upper tract dilatation which in the absence of intact sensation will be entirely asymptomatic. It is imperative therefore that screening programmes which are not based on regular urography include a "plain film" assessment recognising the increased tendency of spinal cord injured patients to form urinary calculi (see below).

Management

The management of upper tract dilatation in spinal cord damaged patients is shown in the two algorithms in Figs. 5.1 and 5.2.

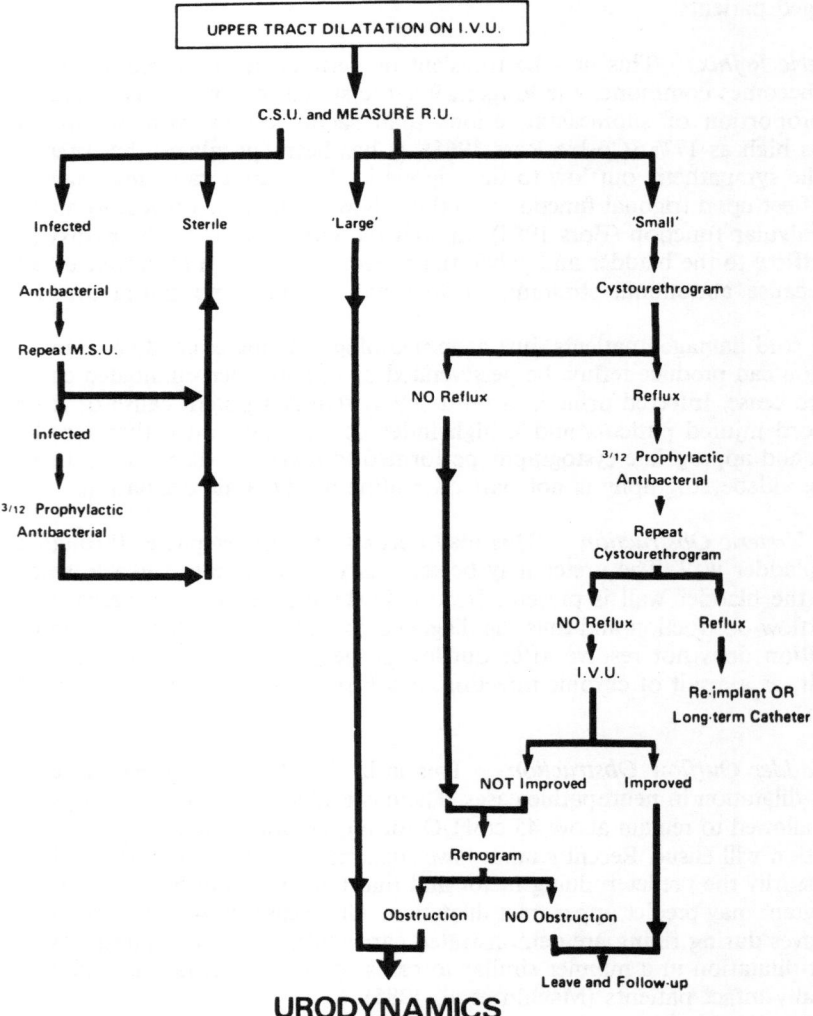

Figure 5.1 Algorithm showing the investigation and management of bilateral upper urinary tract dilatation. (From Gardner et al. 1986.)

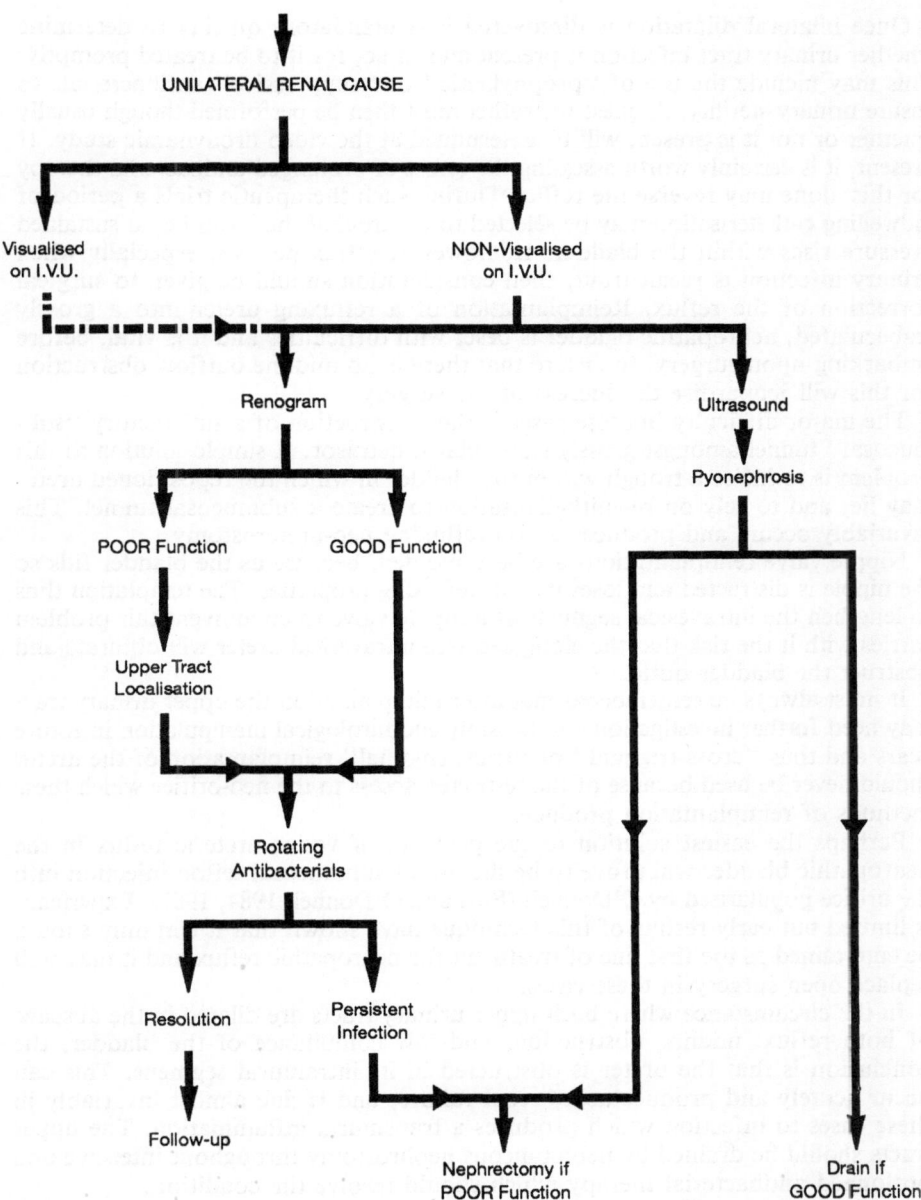

Figure 5.2 Management pathways when a single upper tract is found to be dilated. (From Gardner et al. 1986.)

Bilateral Upper Tract Dilatation

Fig. 5.1 considers bilateral upper tract dilatation, which is commoner than unilateral dilatation.

Once bilateral dilatation is discovered it is mandatory quickly to determine whether urinary tract infection is present and, if so, for it to be treated promptly. This may include the use of "prophylactic" or "suppressive" antibacterials to ensure urinary sterility. A quest for reflux must then be performed though usually whether or not it is present will be determined at the video-urodynamic study. If present, it is certainly worth assessing the effect of prolonged antibacterial therapy for this alone may reverse the reflux. During such therapeutic trials a period of indwelling catheterisation may be selected to ensure that there can be no sustained pressure rises within the bladder. If, however, reflux persists, especially when urinary infection is recalcitrant, then consideration should be given to surgical correction of the reflux. Reimplantation of a refluxing ureter into a grossly trabeculated, neuropathic bladder is beset with difficulties and it is vital, before embarking upon surgery, to ensure that there is no midline outflow obstruction for this will jeopardise the success of the surgery.

The major difficulty in these cases is the construction of a satisfactory "sub-mucosal" tunnel amongst grossly trabeculated detrusor. A simple solution to this problem is to incise a trough within the bladder in which the repositioned ureter may lie, and to rely on re-epithelialisation to create a submucosal tunnel. This invariably occurs and produces a non-refluxing neo-ureterostomy.

Nipple valve reimplantations are best avoided, because as the bladder fills so the nipple is distracted and loses its anti-refluxing properties. The temptation thus to lengthen the intravesical segment of a nipple valve to circumvent this problem carries with it the risk that the elongated free intravesical ureter will obturate and obstruct the bladder outlet.

It must always be remembered that after reimplantation the upper urinary tract may need further investigation and possibly endourological manipulation in future years and thus "cross-trigonal" or "trans-trigonal" reimplantation of the ureter should never be used because of the restricted access to the neo-orifice which these methods of reimplantation produce.

Perhaps the easiest solution to the problem of vesico-ureteric reflux in the neuropathic bladder will prove to be the use of submucosal teflon injection into the orifice popularised by O'Donnell (Puri and O'Donnell 1984, 1987). Experience is limited but early results of this technique have shown that it certainly should be entertained as the first line of treatment for neuropathic reflux and it may well replace open surgery in these cases.

In the circumstance where both upper urinary tracts are dilated in the absence of both reflux, midline obstruction, and low compliance of the bladder, the conclusion is that the ureter is obstructed in its intramural segment. This can occur acutely and produce acute renal failure, and is due almost invariably in these cases to infection which produces a transmural inflammation. The upper tracts should be drained by percutaneous nephrostomy throughout intensive and prolonged antibacterial therapy which should resolve the condition.

In chronic cases, there is no alternative to bilateral ureteric reimplantation to resolve the upper tract obstruction.

Bilateral upper tract dilatation is otherwise due to midline neuropathic bladder outflow obstruction, the management of which is detailed in Chapter 4. Restitution of satisfactory bladder emptying is accompanied in these cases by resolution of the dilatation.

Unilateral Upper Tract Dilatation

Clearly, any of the mechanisms by which bilateral upper tract dilatation is produced may induce just one side to dilate. Therefore the management of a single refluxing ureter, or one that is obstructed in its intramural segment, is as indicated above. Midline obstruction is far less likely to initiate dilatation in one side and not the other but this can occur and thus the bladder outflow should always be investigated completely even on finding of a *unilaterally* dilated upper tract.

There are important considerations when a single side is found to be dilated. If the condition responds to merely intensive antibacterial therapy, then no further intervention is required, though it is important always to follow up the patients carefully. It is a truism, however, that the singly dilated upper tract often loses its function rather more precipitously, perhaps as a result of occult infection. It is important therefore to establish whether infection is present and upper urinary tract infection localisation studies should be considered (Stamey and Pfau 1963; Fairley et al. 1967).

Whilst an intravenous urogram may give the very broadest indication of function, this test is notoriously unreliable as an assessor of function and thus renography is the investigation of choice in these cases, largely to determine renal viability. If infection is localised to a poorly functioning unilaterally dilated upper tract then the system on that side is best removed by nephroureterectomy, rather than to embark upon conservative surgery.

In the severest cases, a pyonephrosis may develop and, interestingly, this can often be diagnosed by ultrasonography. It is always worth draining the kidney, and usually this can be achieved percutaneously. In some cases however, a formal nephrostomy is preferable. In either event, the opportunity is afforded to determine functional recovery. Unlike neurologically intact patients, where it is unusual for a kidney which has developed a severe pyonephrosis to regain useful function, in spinal cord injured patients this is not the case and satisfactory functional return can be anticipated. Why there should be this difference is not known.

In those patients where function does not return, an "interval" nephroureterectomy will be needed and this should be planned at perhaps three to four months. This will allow resolution of the perinephric phlegmon which will facilitate surgery, yet be soon enough for a further pyonephrosis not to develop. In cases where functional recovery does not occur, the nephrostomy drainage tube is removed or, in the authors' experience, usually falls out.

Whatever the cause of the upper tract dilatation and whether it is uni- or bilateral, those patients in whom it has occurred must be followed up with the utmost diligence for the frailty of the urinary tract has been revealed and its vulnerability demonstrated. By careful urological surveillance and prompt intervention when indicated, the threat to their lives from this aspect of the spinal injury can be lifted.

Stones

Upper Urinary Tract Calculi

Approximately 6% of spinal cord damaged patients will develop upper urinary tract calculi, compared with 2% in the general population. The sex distribution of patients with stones in the order of 5: 1 (Gardner et al. 1985) reflects the ratio of males to females who sustain spinal cord injury, which contrasts with the general population where stones are twice as common in males between the second to sixth decade.

Although many calculi are diagnosed within two years of injury, over two-thirds present after this time, indicating that recumbency is not the sole aetiological factor. Infection is important in the genesis of calculi in spinal cord damaged patients and, as in neurologically intact patients, the presence of a *Proteus* species urinary infection carries with it a significantly increased risk of stone development. Whether or not urinary infection is present, however, at no stage does the risk of stone development in spinal injured patients disappear.

Biochemical investigation seldom reveals any metabolic abnormality and hyperparathyroidism is rather rarer a cause of stone disease than it is in the normal population.

There is no clear relationship between the incidence of upper urinary tract calculi and the neurological level. They rarely occur in patients with lesions below L1, but the significance of this observation is unknown.

Approximately 80% of stones are discovered by routine radiographic follow-up. Recurring urinary tract infection accounts for the majority of the remainder. Renal or ureteric pain is extremely uncommon, even in patients with lesions at T11 or below. Hypertension, haematuria or increased peripheral somatic spasm are rare presenting features which should raise the index of suspicion and provoke a careful search for upper tract calculi which can sometimes be difficult to see at plain radiography because of gaseous gut distension or constipation. Some patients may develop large calculi with great rapidity indicating the hazard associated with infrequent urological follow-up.

The majority of upper tract calculi found in spinal injured patients are small and single but multiple or bilateral stones may be present at initial presentation to the Spinal Injuries Unit soon after injury. Whereas 10% of stones in the general population are radiolucent only 4% are found to be so in spinal cord damaged patients.

Infection, obstruction and permanent loss of renal function are common complications, perhaps because of the paucity of symptoms which are provoked and thus early treatment of calculi in this population is vital.

Management

Prior to the recent development in endourological and lithotriptor technology (Segura et al. 1983; Chaussy and Schmiedt 1983; 1984; Lee et al. 1985) a conservative approach to upper tract calculi was often adopted. This was justified because of potential hazards due either to operative difficulties, such as inaccessibility due to spinal deformity, or possible postoperative morbidity in patients who do not have normal cardioregulatory responses, and particularly in tetraplegic patients who have borderline respiratory function. No doubt several patients who were managed by this "wait and see" approach suffered either serious infections or significant deterioration in renal function.

Reticence regarding active intervention is thus no longer acceptable and all the modern modalities of stone management (Bush et al. 1984; Brannen et al. 1985; Marberger et al. 1985; Mayo et al. 1985) should be available to spinal injured cases. Modern percutaneous lithotriptors, either ultrasonic or electrohydraulic, can disintegrate most calculi speedily and without morbidity (Clayman et al. 1983; Segura et al. 1983; Wickham et al. 1983; Elder et al 1984; Lee et al. 1985). Rigid ureterorenoscopy allows access to the upper ureter for endoscopic extraction of calculi and this lowers the threshold for intervention for high ureteric stones (Ford et al 1983; Huffman et al. 1983; Watson et al. 1983).

The indications for intervention are thus when the stone obstructs, or threatens to obstruct any part of the upper urinary tract from the infundibulum of the calyx to the lower end of the ureter; if there is recurring infection; when renal parenchymal integrity is threatened; if the calculus increases in size; and finally, and perhaps rather more contentiously, if there is a risk of poor compliance by the patient on a follow-up programme.

Transurethral endoscopic and percutaneous endoscopic surgery can safely be performed in spinal cord injury centres, but extracorporeal lithotripsy demands that the patient be moved to a stone centre. Impaired cardiovascular and respiratory function, vulnerable skin and propensity to spasm in many spinal cord damaged patients render extracorporeal lithotripsy perhaps less appropriate, and a careful balance must be weighed to determine the best treatment option for a given stone in the light of these considerations (Finlayson and Thomas 1984; Weber et al. 1984).

The current options of management of upper tract calculi are shown in Figs. 5.3, 5.4 and 5.5.

Bladder Calculi

The majority of intravesical calculi found in spinal cord injured patients originate as encrustations around retaining catheter balloons and progress to become "eggshell" stones. These may be detected radiologically at an early stage but in some patients become substantial in size, multiple, and laminated in character. These laminations render them susceptible to lithotripsy either with a classical lithotrite or by electrohydraulic lithotripsy, which has become the method of choice for these calculi.

Other bladder calculi can be found in relation to persistent bladder neck obstruction in both males and females in the absence of catheters. They tend to be of firmer consistency yet usually are still readily treatable by endovesical lithotripsy. It is indeed exceptionally unusual to have to resort to open lithotomy for bladder calculus in spinal cord injured patients but this operation will occasionally be necessary when, often because of inattention to urological surveillance, a bladder stone becomes too large or too hard to be dealt with endoscopically.

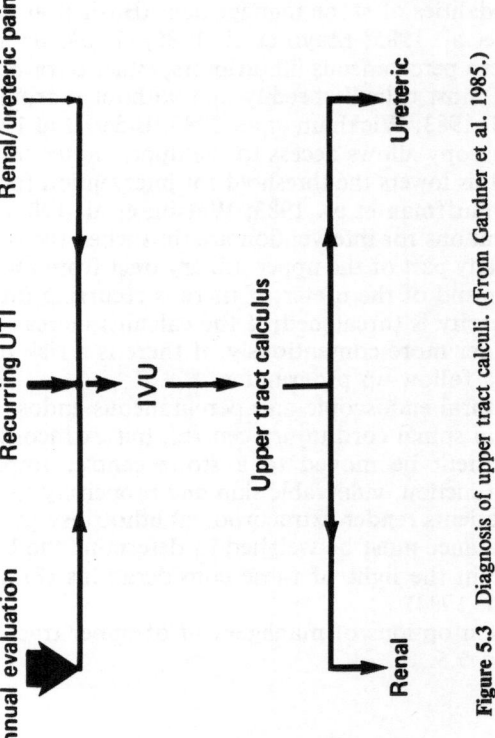

Figure 5.3 Diagnosis of upper tract calculi. (From Gardner et al. 1985.)

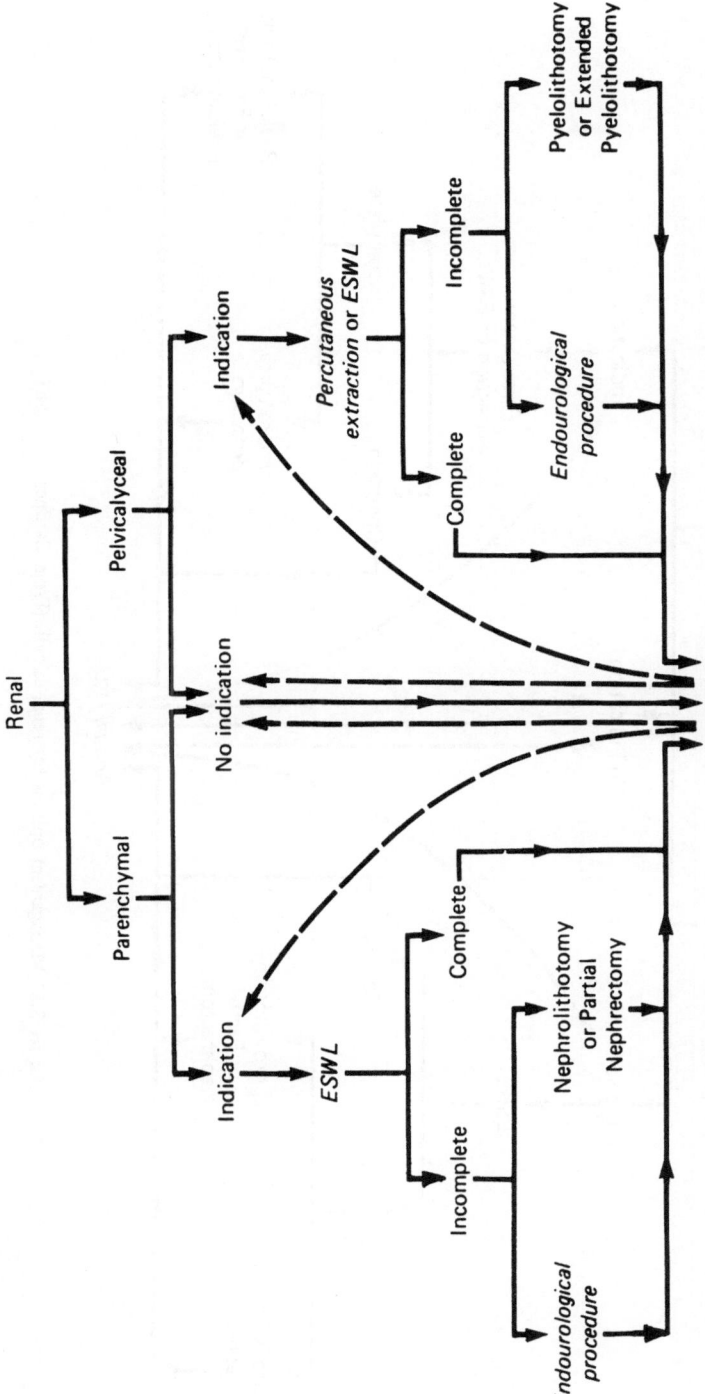

Figure 5.4 The management of ureteric calculi utilising endourological procedures. (From Gardner et al. 1985.)

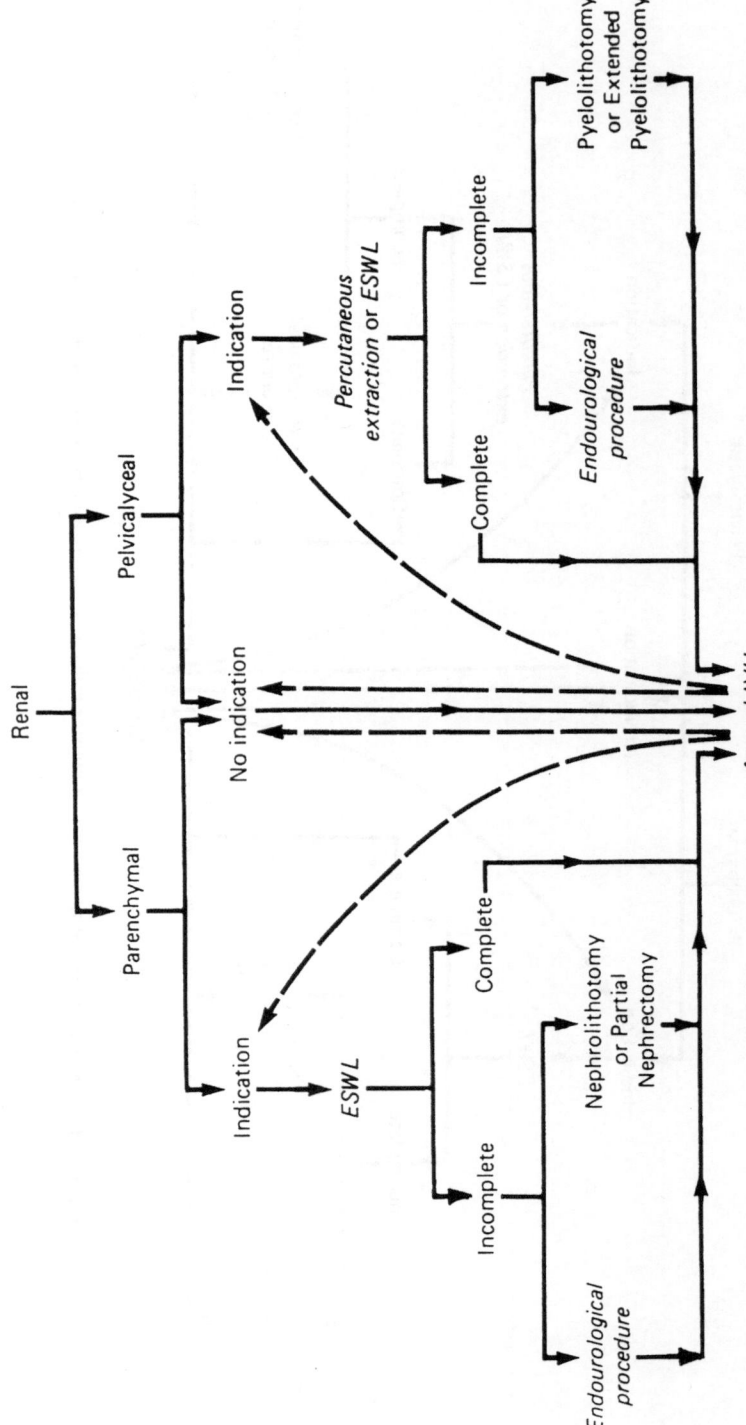

Figure 5.5 Management options for renal calculi. (From Gardner et al. 1985.)

References

Bors E (1954) Bladder disturbances and management of patients with injury to the spinal cord. J Int Coll Surg 21: 513–527

Brannen GE, Bush WH, Correa RJ et al. (1985) Kidney stone removal: percutaneous versus surgical lithotomy. J Urol 113: 6–12

Breithaupt DJ, Jousse AT, Wynne-Jones M (1961) Late cause of death and life expectancy in paraplegia. Can Med Assoc J 85: 73–77

Bush WH, Brannen GE, Gibbons RP et al. (1984) Radiation exposure to patient and urologist during percutaneous nephrostolithotomy. J Urol 132: 1148–1152

Chaussy C, Schmiedt E (1983) Shock wave treatment for stones in the upper urinary tract. Urol Clin North Am 10: 743–750

Chaussy C, Schmiedt E (1984) Four years experience with extracorporeal shock wave lithotripsy (ESWL) in Munich. J Urol 131: 264a

Clayman RV, Surya V, Miller RP et al. (1983) Percutaneous nephrolithotomy. An approach to branched and staghorn renal calculi. JAMA 250: 73–75

Cosbie Ross J (1965) Vesico-ureteric reflux in the neurogenic bladder. Br J Surg 52: 164–167

Elder JS, Gibbons RP, Bush WH (1984) Ultrasonic lithotripsy of a large staghorn calculus. J Urol 131: 1152–1154

Fairley KF, Bond AG, Brown RB et al. (1967) Simple test to determine the site of urinary tract infection. Lancet 2: 427

Finlayson B, Thomas WC Jr (1984) Extracorporeal shock wave lithotripsy. Ann Intern Med 101(3): 387–389

Ford TF, Watson GM, Wickham JEA (1983) Transurethral ureteroscopic retrieval of ureteric stones. Br J Urol 55: 626–628

Gardner BP, Parsons KF, Soni BM, Krishnan KR (1985) The management of upper tract calculi in spinal cord damaged patients. Paraplegia 23: 371–378

Gardner BP, Parsons KF, Machin DG, Galloway A, Krishnan KR (1986) Urological management of spinal cord damaged patients: a clinical algorithm. Paraplegia 24: 138–147

Geisler WO, Jousse AT, Wynne-Jones M (1977) Survival in traumatic transverse myelitis. Paraplegia 14: 262–275

Geisler WO, Jousse AT, Wynne-Jones M, Briethaupt DJ (1983) Survival in traumatic spinal cord injury. Paraplegia 21: 364–373

Huffman JL, Bagley DM, Schoenberg HW, Lyon ES (1983) Transurethral removal of large ureteral and renal pelvic calculi using ureteroscopic ultrasonic lithotripsy. J Urol 130: 31–34

Jousse AT, Wynne-Jones M, Breithaupt DJ (1968) A follow-up study of life expectancy and mortality in traumatic transverse myelitis. Can Med Assoc J 98: 770–772

Lee WJ, Loh G, Smith AD et al. (1985) Percutaneous extraction of renal stones: experience in 100 patients. AJR 144: 451–455

Machin DG, Gardner BP, Woolfenden KA et al. (1985) A physiological approach to the investigation of chronic urinary retention. Br J Urol 57: 141–144

Marberger M, Stackl W, Hruby W, Kroiss A (1985) Late sequelae of ultrasonic lithotripsy of renal calculi. J Urol 133: 170–173

Mayo ME, Kriegger JN, Rudd TG (1985) Effect of percutaneous nephrostolithotomy on renal function. J Urol 133: 167–169

O'Reilly PH, Shields RA, Testa HJ (eds) (1986) Nuclear medicine in urology, 2nd edn. Butterworths, London

Puri P, O'Donnell B (1984) Correction of experimentally produced vesicoureteric reflux in the piglet by intravesical injection of teflon. Br Med J 289: 5–7

Puri P, O'Donnell B (1987) Endoscopic correction of grades IV and V primary vesicoureteric reflux: six to 30 month follow-up in 42 ureters. J Pediatr Surg 22: 1087–1091

Segura JW (1984) Endourology. Review article. J Urol 132: 167–169

Segura JW, Patterson DE, LeRoy AJ et al. (1983) Percutaneous lithotripsy. J Urol 130: 1051–1054

Stamey TA, Pfau A (1963) Some functional, pathologic, bacteriologic and chemotherapeutic characteristics of unilateral pyelonephritis in man: II. Bacteriologic and chemotherapeutic characteristics. Invest Urol 1: 162

Watson GM, Wickham JEA, Mills TN et al. (1983) Laser fragmentation of renal calculi. Br J Urol 55: 613–616

Weber W, Chaussy C, Madler C et al. (1984) Cardiocirculatory changes during anaesthesia for
  extracorporeal shock wave lithotripsy. J Urol 131: 246a
Wickham JEA, Kellett MJ, Miller RA (1983) Elective percutaneous nephrolithotomy in 50 patients:
  an analysis of the technique, results and complications. J Urol 129: 904–906

Chapter 6

Urinary Tract Infection

P.C. Ryan and J.M. Fitzpatrick

Introduction

The outlook for patients following traumatic injury to the spinal cord has changed dramatically in the past 70 years and this has been due in large degree to improvements in the prevention and management of urosepsis. Earlier this century, the mortality in patients who had suffered spinal cord injury was 80% and, in the majority of cases, death resulted from infection of the urinary tract (Thompson-Walker 1917). Today, mortality in acutely injured patients is less than 5% and this usually results from respiratory failure, multiple injuries or pulmonary emboli (Grundy et al. 1986). There are two principal reasons for the improved prognosis in these patients. First, the realisation that the spinal cord injured patient is acutely unable to drain the urinary tract and is therefore prone to bacterial colonisation of urine resulted in artificial drainage becoming a priority in the acutely injured patient, with consequent diminution in the incidence of fulminant sepsis. Second, the development of potent antimicrobial agents has meant that infection, where it occurs, can be treated and the resulting renal failure prevented.

As management in the acute phase of injury has improved, more and more patients have survived the initial stages after injury. The aims in management of these patients have therefore changed from drainage of the urinary tract at any cost to the current goals where protection of the upper tracts from damage due to back pressure or infection, urinary continence with catheter freedom and maximal prevention of sepsis are the priorities. Improvements in management have been aided by the development of better catheters in terms of design and materials used; improved diagnostic techniques including imaging, urodynamic and microbiological analysis and the use of recent generation antimicrobials with a true understanding of their indications and drawbacks.

The most frequent complication following spinal cord injury is still urinary tract infection (Young 1982) but this condition persists as a recurrent clinical problem with significant morbidity, rather than a life-threatening event in the majority of spinal cord injured patients. Nevertheless, a higher incidence of urosepsis is associated with mortality after spinal injury (Webb et al. 1984).

Pathogenesis of Urinary Tract Infection Following Spinal Cord Injury

Normal Defences

In describing the pathogenesis of urinary tract infection following spinal cord injury, one should first consider the natural defences of the urinary tract against infection. The system is exposed at the penile urethral meatus to the external environment and an epithelial surface protects the urethra, bladder, ureters and kidneys against invasion of the body tissues by organisms present within the urine. Under normal circumstances, urine is continuously produced by the kidney and a constant antegrade flow maintains the tract free of pathogenic organisms. Urine is continuously propelled from the upper tract into the bladder by active and passive transport within the ureter and reflux from the bladder into the ureter is prevented by a valve-like mechanism at the uretero-vesical junction. Urine is then stored within the bladder and voided intermittently through the urethra during normal micturition. In this way, stasis of urine which might act as a medium for multiplication of organisms is prevented. A further defence within the bladder against infection is the production of IgA by the urothelial lining.

Classification of Spinal Cord Injury

Transport of urine within the upper urinary tract by ureteric peristalsis occurs involuntarily and without neural reflex activity. The act of micturition involves voluntary stimulus from the cerebral cortex conducted down the spinal cord and, in addition, autonomic reflexes which are mediated principally by parasympathetic nerves. These voluntary and reflex impulses are co-ordinated in a spinal cord centre which is located at the level of the T12–L1 vertebrae.

Spinal cord injury can broadly be subdivided into upper motor neurone and lower motor neurone lesions. An upper motor neurone lesion occurs when the spinal cord is damaged above the level of the spinal micturition centre, resulting in loss of influence from higher centres but intact bladder reflexes. When injury to the conus, cauda equina, or pelvic nerves causes a lower motor neurone lesion, the bladder is also devoid of reflex neurone control. In practice, the division between these lesions is by no means clear cut (Grundy et al. 1986), as lesions of the spinal cord are often incomplete and, furthermore, ischaemia distal to a lesion high in the spinal cord can cause extension of injury. The initial response of the bladder following spinal cord injury is a period of spinal shock, where no active function occurs in the lower urinary tract. During this phase the bladder is atonic and the external urethral sphincter is in a state of contraction which cannot be voluntarily relaxed (O'Flynn 1974). The result is that drainage of the lower urinary tract is acutely cut off and retention occurs, with the risk of bacterial colonisation. The priority in urological management of spinal shock is to establish bladder drainage as soon as possible. One method (probably the preferable method) of achieving this end is to perform intermittent catheterisation of the bladder with a narrow gauge under aseptic conditions at a frequency which prevents the bladder from overdistending beyond 500 ml (Guttman and Frankel 1966). Fluid intake is restricted to 1500 ml per 24 hours. Alternatively, patients may be managed by suprapubic catherisation from the time of injury with the advantages that there is no urethral trauma, a high fluid intake can be maintained and there is less of a burden on the attending personnel. Continuous catheterisation can also be achieved using an indwelling urethral catheter during spinal shock and manual expression of the atonic bladder has also been used during this period, but neither of these methods has any advantage over intermittent catheterisation or suprapubic continuous drainage.

The second phase of management begins as soon as spontaneous activity within the bladder returns and a re-education process attempts to achieve balanced bladder function. During this period of bladder retraining drainage may be achieved once again by intermittent catherisation, indwelling urethral or suprapubic catheter or manual expression, the latter technique often combined with attempts to stimulate reflex bladder emptying.

Eventually, a steady state is reached where the patient is successfully emptying his bladder by one of the aforementioned techniques. The acontractile bladder due to a lower motor neurone lesion is best treated in both sexes by self intermittent catheterisation (SIC) with or without the use of imipramine to suppress spontaneous bladder contractions. Alternatively, these patients may use manual expression in the suprapubic area to empty their bladder, which technique in males may be combined with phenoxybenzamine to relax the external sphincter or an external sphincterotomy. The upper motor neurone bladder which can undergo reflex emptying can be managed in males by suprapubic tapping with manual expression while the patient wears a condom to collect the urine. An external sphincterotomy may be needed in these patients if the bladder outlet is obstructive. Alternatively, if upper limb function allows, SIC can be combined with anticholinergic agents or imipramine, either of which will suppress bladder contraction and facilitate acceptable bladder capacity. A final option in these patients is the use of an indwelling catheter.

In female patients with an upper motor neurone bladder, the Credé manoeuvre has been shown to be a satisfactory means of emptying the bladder in a significant number of patients (Grainger et al. 1988). Clean SIC is an acceptable alternative. The choice of management in patients with upper motor neurone lesions will, of course, depend on the extent to which upper limb function is preserved.

Self intermittent catheterisation or manual expression will not be possible in patients where upper limb function is absent or very poor. Appropriate application of bladder drainage options has been greatly aided by the use of urodynamic investigations (Rossier and Bushra 1979). As each technique has its own implications regarding sepsis, patients must be carefully and properly assessed and the optimal choice for bladder drainage made.

Pathogenic Factors in Urosepsis

What then are the specific factors that predispose to urinary tract sepsis following spinal cord injury? Urinary stasis occurs when bladder emptying by whatever means fails to empty the bladder completely, with a consequent residual urine. The critical volume of residual urine requiring intervention is greater than 150 ml. The residual urine does not in itself cause infection, but when contamination results from the introduction of catheters or the continuing application of condom drainage, residual urine acts as a culture medium or sump for bacterial colonisation (O'Grady and Catell 1966; Kyle 1968). It has been shown that the incidence of bacteriuria is proportional to the volume of residual urine occurring in spinal cord injury patients (Merritt 1981). In addition, restriction of fluids in patients who are performing SIC increases the instance of sepsis (Pearman 1976), probably because fluid restriction promotes urinary stasis.

Overdistension of the bladder is a potential risk, particularly in the spinal shocked patient where drainage is not adequately maintained and this has a number of effects on defences against infection. Decreased elimination of bacteria and electron microscopic evidence of damage to mucosal integrity were observed in experimentally overdistended bladders (Lloyd-Davies and Hinman 1971).

Furthermore, fibrosis is induced within the bladder wall with loss of contractility (Bradley et al. 1967; Lloyd-Davies et al. 1970; Gibbon 1974) and sacculation also occurs (Gibbon 1974). Other causes of overdistension are detrusor-sphincter dyssynergia, which occurs in a significant proportion of spinal cord injured patients, and also the application of manual expression as a means of bladder emptying (Pearman and England 1973). Bladder overdistension also gives rise to delay in return of reflex bladder activity after the initial period of spinal shock.

Reflex bladder contraction in the presence of bladder outlet obstruction causes a raised intravesical pressure and this characteristically occurs in the bladder associated with an upper motor neurone lesion particularly when there is detrusor-sphincter dyssynergia. The bladder hypertrophies to overcome increased outflow resistance and as a result urine refluxes into the upper urinary tract causing renal damage from back pressure. Vesico-ureteric reflux also causes recurrent ascending pyelonephritis when the bladder contains infected urine and, although this condition is reversible if residual urine and infection are subsequently prevented (Gibbon 1974), renal scarring with chronic pyelonephritis may result if the condition is not adequately treated. Infection per se is thought to cause vesico-ureteric reflux by some workers (Kyle 1968; Silver 1974) but there is some disagreement about this (Gross and Liebowitz 1981). The mechanism by which infection might cause reflux is thought to be oedema and ulceration within the wall of the bladder in the presence of cystitis, causing incontinence of the uretero-vesical valve mechanism.

There are a number of factors contributing to the formation of urinary tract calculi in spinal injury. Urinary stasis within the bladder and upper tracts and infected urine, particularly with urea-splitting organisms such as *Proteus* (Nikakhta et al. 1981; Vargus et al. 1982), both predispose to calculus formation. Spinal cord patients are often recumbent and the resultant hypercalciuria promotes calculus formation.

Reflux of infected urine is an important factor in renal stone formation and it has been shown that the incidence of renal calculi is proportional not to the method of drainage but to the rate of sepsis (De Vivo et al. 1984; Kohli and

Lamid 1986). Other mechanisms causing formation of calculi within the bladder include pubic hairs introduced during intermittent self catheterisation or egg shell calculi which form on the balloon of an indwelling catheter (Grundy et al. 1986). Urinary tract calculi are more common in upper motor neurone compared to lower motor neurone lesions and a close correlation exists between the occurrence of urinary tract calculi and mortality rates in spinal cord injured patients (Sharpe et al. 1971). There are conflicting data regarding the incidence of urinary tract calculi in spinal cord injured patients: an overall incidence of 6% is quoted (Anderson 1986), but other workers have suggested that the incidence of urolithiasis is 9% in SIC patients alone (Berard et al. 1985), while other studies have consistently shown an incidence of 8% overall (De Vivo et al. 1984; Comarr et al. 1962). A series of 893 spinal cord injury patients was reviewed in order to establish risk factors for the formation of renal calculi (Kohli and Lamid 1986). In this series, level of spinal injury, completeness of spinal cord lesion, method of urinary drainage or presence of ureteric reflux all seemed unrelated to the incidence of renal stone formation, nor was the absence of physical activity a risk factor. There was correlation between sepsis, positive urine culture and the incidence of renal tract calculi. Clearly, infection and calculous disease are two closely related complications of spinal cord injury and are combined synergistically as a mechanism of damage to the urinary tract in spinal cord injured patients.

Insertion of bladder catheters and application of condoms are important mechanisms for the development and persistence of urinary tract infections. As mentioned above, poor bladder emptying with residual urine is not in itself a cause of infection, but rather a reservoir for infection introduced by bladder catheters. It has been shown that one source of infection of the bladder in spinal cord injured patients is the anterior urethra (Stickler et al. 1970) and insertion of a catheter into the bladder per urethram causes spread of these organisms. If the catheter is indwelling, it acts as a foreign body which potentiates infection and makes it difficult to eradicate (Hardy 1968).

Another factor is that an indwelling catheter, particularly if the balloon is inflated, may not empty the bladder completely, leaving a residue of infected urine. This is particularly true in the recumbent patient where the tip of the balloon catheter will not lie in the most dependent part of the bladder. Urinary tract infection can be particularly difficult to eradicate even after removal of an indwelling urethral catheter and one theory as to the source of such persistent infection is that an indwelling catheter is associated with chronic obstruction of the urethral and prostatic glands, which become colonised with bacteria (Kyle 1968). Indwelling catheters also have local pressure and irritative effects. Trauma caused by passage of catheters or instruments, with the possibility of a false passage, also contribute to the development of sepsis and the frequency of instrumentation of the lower urinary tract is related to the incidence of urinary tract infection (Hardy 1968; Peatfield et al. 1983; Montgomerie et al. 1986). Local complications of indwelling catheters include urethritis and epididymitis which can be related to either local obstruction at the ejaculatory duct or obstruction to outflow by a catheter-induced stricture. Seminal vesiculitis, peri-urethral abscess with subsequent fistula formation (Kyle 1968), urethral diverticulum and perivesical abscess (Ascoli 1968) are other catheter-associated problems. Of these, infection of the seminal vesicles secondary to catheterisation can be particularly difficult to eradicate (Kyle 1968).

The source or nidus of infection in spinal cord injured patients who have urinary tract sepsis which proves difficult or impossible to eradicate is of particular pathogenic significance, as management techniques which contribute to a longstanding source of infection should be avoided. As outlined above, if the urethral mucosal glands or prostatic ducts are chronically obstructed by the presence of an indwelling urethral catheter, colonisation of these glands by bacteria may be difficult or impossible to treat and may act as a reservoir for infection. Alternatively, the wall of the bladder which has been overdistended or chronically irritated by the presence of an indwelling catheter with concomitant sepsis, may act as a nidus for infection. The wearing of a condom should not be forgotten as a source of sepsis as the external drainage system is very commonly colonised with infecting organisms and urinary tract infection may result (Hirsh et al. 1979).

As in all infective processes, the balance between pathogen and host resistance is crucial. The level of resitance to infection in spinal cord injured patients depends on the severity of injury and the degree to which the major organ systems in the body are compromised. Some workers believe that host resistance factors and the mechanics of bladder emptying are more important than inoculation of potentially infecting organisms in the bladder where the prevention of urinary tract infections in neurogenic bladder patients is concerned (Lapides et al. 1972; Lapides 1973). The patient may have urinary tract colonisation without pathological effects if the virulence of the organism is low and host resistance is maintained at an optimal level by adequate nutritional and haematological care and maintenance of maximal mobility (Kyle 1968). Regarding microbial virulence, the degree to which antibiotics are administered will determine to what extent resistant organisms are selected out and also the survival of commensal organisms, whose role in the suppression of pathogens cannot be underestimated.

A variety of infecting organisms are reported in different series but one common theme is that they are often organisms which would not cause infection in the normal bladder, such as *Staphylococcus epidermidis* or *Candida albicans* (Anderson 1986; Pearman 1971). These opportunistic pathogens are allowed to colonise the urine because of immunosuppression, leukopenia or the removal of normal flora as a result of broad-spectrum antibiotics (Lindan 1978). In female patients undergoing SIC, the most common infecting organism was *E. coli* with a lesser instance of *Proteus, Klebsiella, Pseudomonas, Serratia* or *Citrobacter* (Joiner and Lindan 1982). In a series of 59 patients admitted to a spinal injury unit with sterile urine and treated by intermittent catheterisation, the first infections detected in 56 patients were *Klebsiella aerogenes* ($n = 19$), *Streptococcus faecalis* ($n = 6$), *Pseudomonas pyocyanea* ($n = 6$), *Proteus* ($n = 14$), *E. freundii* ($n = 1$), *Providencia* ($n = 4$), *E. coli* ($n = 3$) and *Aerobacter clocae* ($n = 3$) and many of these were nosocomial infections (Silver 1974). When prophylactic antibiotic agents were compared with no treatment in a series of 151 male patients the infecting organisms detected included *E. coli, Pseudomonas* (most commonly), *Enterococcus, Serratia narcescens, Klebsiella* and *Proteus mirabilis* (Kuhlemeier et al. 1985).

The role of *Pseudomonas* in spinal cord injured patients is of particular interest and may, indeed, bear close relation to the significance of other so-called opportunistic pathogens. *P. aeruginosa* is a pathogen in immunocompromised hosts, for example patients with malignant disease, but rarely if ever proliferates in the presence of normal host resistance to infection. The success of this organism as an opportunist and a coloniser is due in part to the production of antibiotic substances which suppress other flora (Bouchard 1989). One group of workers have records of patients showing repeated isolations of *Pseudomonas* but without any symptoms or evidence of renal damage in renal function studies and suggest that *Pseudomonas*, by virtue of antibiotic production, may act as a "keeper at the gate" in the bladder of spinal cord injured patients, preventing infection by pathogens (Lindan and Joiner 1984).

The urethra and perineum of patients with spinal cord injury are frequently colonised by *Pseudomonas* and this may explain why *Pseudomonas* bacteriuria has been commonly detected in these patients (Montgomerie and Morrow 1980; Gilmore et al. 1982).

A factor in the spread of hospital organisms is the presence of a large number of patients with infected urine on a ward, since it is difficult for the ward staff to manage a large number of catheterisations and maintain sterility (Silver 1974). Although there is a significant incidence of opportunistic pathogens of questionable virulence in the spinal cord injured patient, Gram-negative sepsis was the predominant cause of death in patients who had spinal cord injury and consequent end-stage renal disease (Barton et al. 1984), and the dangers of infection with Gram-negative pathogens must never be underestimated.

A factor which must be emphasised in describing the pathogenesis of urosepsis in spinal cord injured patients and which must not be overlooked in the clinical management is the potentially asymptomatic progress of disease. Depending on the level of the lesion, the spinal cord injured patient may have inadequate or absent sensation within the urinary tract (Wyndaele et al. 1983; Anderson 1986; Grundy and Russell 1986) and sepsis or the complication thereof may occur without the warning of early symptoms. Other infective complications not mentioned above which can occur in spinal cord injured patients include acute or chronic prostatitis, bladder diverticula, pyocystis, acute or chronic pyelonephritis and urethral stricture.

Renal failure, the worst of all complications and the symbol of failed management in spinal cord injured patients, may involve amyloidosis as a pathological finding and is related to the development of back pressure transmitted from the lower urinary tract. However, the most significant cause of renal failure appears to be urinary tract infection and its associated complications (Kyle 1968; Barton et al. 1984; Cardenas and Mayo 1987).

Clinical Management

Overview

It is clear that the pathogenesis of urinary tract infection in spinal cord injured patients is complex, when compared to the normal individual, and that many factors are involved. The objectives in management are to preserve renal function by preventing sepsis and back pressure and, at the same time, achieve optimal quality of life. Adequate drainage of the bladder, preferably without indwelling foreign material, should be maintained so that there is no reservoir for bacterial colonisation or overdistension of the bladder. Optimal host resistance is essential and the aim should be to prevent rather than treat infection and its complications (Wyndaele 1987). There are three phases in the management of the spinal cord injured patient: initial spinal shock, bladder re-education or training and follow-up. Each of these phases requires specific types of management and regular monitoring of renal tract function and bacterial invasion is mandatory.

Bladder Drainage

Acute

Immediately following spinal cord injury a period of spinal shock exists where the bladder is atonic. This causes acute retention of urine in approximately 80% of spinal cord injured patients (O'Flynn 1974). It is essential that these patients are catheterised immediately (Gardiner et al. 1986) to prevent the sequelae of overdistension of the bladder. The dilemma is which type of bladder drainage technique to use.

(a) Intermittent Catheterisation. Perhaps the single greatest advance in the management of spinal cord injured patients has been the introduction by Sir Ludwig Guttmann of intermittent catheterisation as a means of acute management of the shocked bladder (Guttman and Frankel 1966). The advantages of intermittent catheterisation from the microbiological point of view are considerable. The bladder is emptied efficiently without any indwelling foreign material and a sterile technique can be used to perform this procedure. The technique is performed as frequently as is necessary to ensure that the residual urine is less than 500 ml, thus preventing overdistension.

The catheter is slowly withdrawn from the bladder so that complete emptying is achieved. The fact that the bladder is intermittently filled means that a normal capacity is maintained and this can be varied by altering the frequency of intermittent catheterisation and/or volume of oral fluids. Disadvantages of this technique include urethral trauma resulting from frequent passage of the catheter and restriction of oral fluids to less than 1500 ml per 24 hours which is usually maintained in order to lessen the burden of frequent catheterisation on medical personnel. The results from this technique are excellent in terms of the incidence of bacteriuria (Guttman and Frankel 1966; Walsh 1968; Pearman 1971; O'Flynn 1974; Wyndaele et al. 1985; Grundy and Russell 1986; Gardiner et al. 1986; Anderson 1986; Wyndaele 1987). A further advantage is that patients who have been treated initially by indwelling catheters can be converted to intermittent catheterisation and results of this management show that pre-existing infection rates can be markedly improved (Miller 1971; Ott and Rossier 1971). It has also been observed that results are similar when intermittent catheterisation is performed by trained nursing personnel compared to doctors (Ott and Rossier 1971).

(b) Urethral Indwelling Catheterisation. The acutely shocked bladder can also be drained by the insertion of a urethral indwelling catheter. This has the advantage that urine is continually drained without necessitating frequent attendance by medical personnel or trauma to the lower urinary tract associated with intermittent catheterisation. In addition, a high fluid intake can be maintained which prevents infection and calculi (O'Flynn 1974; Grundy and Russell 1986). Indeed it may be recommended that indwelling catheterisation be continued if urinary infection has become established until the urine is cleared of infection and debris. A 12F or 14F Foley catheter with a 5 ml balloon should be used. A latex catheter should be

changed weekly but silicone may be retained for up to 6 weeks. When a patient is very ill, or has multiple injuries, urethral indwelling catheterisation may be the method of choice (O'Flynn 1974). The disadvantages of this technique are that all patients will become infected if the catheter is left in for long enough (O'Flynn 1974) and that the incidence of complications associated with indwelling catheters is unacceptably high (Ascoli 1968; Guttman 1976), but it has been correctly pointed out that these complications may be preferable to renal failure from an inadequately drained bladder (Comarr 1961; Gibbon 1966: Cooke and Smith 1968).

(c) Suprapubic Indwelling Catheterisation. The passage of a fine-bore suprapubic catheter also has the advantage of allowing a high fluid intake to be maintained without any trauma to the urethra. The catheter can be clamped intermittently to increase bladder capacity and this technique has an advantage in young individuals where diuresis following spinal cord injury may make intermittent catheterisation impractical (Anderson 1986). This technique also causes less demand on medical personnel and is applicable to the very ill or severely injured patient.

This technique has been increasingly used in the acute management of spinal cord injury (Grundy and Russell 1986). The main disadvantage is the risk of catheter blockage (Grundy et al. 1983). Suprapubic indwelling catheters are cheap and infection rates are similar to those related to intermittent urethral catheterisation (Grundy et al. 1983).

(d) Manual Expression. Bladder emptying in the acute phase of spinal shock by manual expression has been described (Golden 1968) and might seem to have the advantage that it prevents the need for bladder catheterisation. However, when the technique was critically assessed in six patients it was found to be unsatisfactory, resulting in dilatation of the upper urinary tracts, cystitis and increased incidence of deep vein thrombosis (Smith et al. 1972). It was later agreed that this technique is contraindicated in the spinal shocked bladder (Pearman and England 1973; Rossier and Bushra 1979).

Re-education

As the period of spinal shock comes to an end, spontaneous activity is regained in the bladder. The next objective is to establish balanced bladder function, where the bladder is adequately drained of urine, if possible without the application of catheterisation. Pharmacological treatment with alpha-adrenergic blockers, anticholinergic agents or imipramine can be of considerable benefit (Wein 1984). A satisfactory residual urine will have been attained when there is no dilatation of the upper tracts, the urine is sterile, and there is no difficulty in voiding (Gardner et al. 1986). Once the patient can sit up, intermittent catheterisation by hospital personnel can be converted to SIC where the patient catheterises himself or herself with a 12F or 14F Nelaton catheter (Grundy et al. 1986). When the daily residual urine is below 80 ml on three consecutive occasions catheterisation can be discontinued and this usually occurs 6–12 weeks following injury.

Alternatively, or in addition, suprapubic tapping in those patients with an upper motor neurone lesion or suprapubic compression, with or without abdominal straining in lower motor neurone lesions, are methods used to restore regular bladder emptying (Optiz 1984). Intermittent catheterisation as a means of bladder retraining achieves a functional reflex bladder in an average of 78 days (Perkash 1974). Other workers believe that the most effective means of stimulating bladder activity is repeated sharp suprapubic tapping (Glahn 1970). Whatever method of drainage is used during the period of bladder training, there is no doubt that intermittent distension, either by intermittent catheterisation or by intermittent clamping of an indwelling catheter, is an important stimulus in the return of bladder contractile activity (Bradley et al. 1963; Jameson 1969; Gibbon 1974).

Long-term Management

The aims in the spinal shock and re-education phases of rehabilitation are to avoid infection, protect the upper tract and provide conditions for the optimal return of bladder function. Once a steady state is reached, preservation of continence and social acceptability are additional priorities. SIC is a technique capable of achieving all of these objectives and it is applicable to both upper motor neurone and lower motor neurone lesion (Grundy and Russell 1986). Renal function with continence is preserved (Kass et al. 1981) and the incidence of bacteriuria with fever is less than in patients who are treated by an indwelling catheter (Cardenas and Mayo 1987). Follow-up of patients on SIC has shown that a well-balanced bladder is achieved within 260 days for self catheterisation patients compared to 530 days for other patients. No increased incidence of meatal stenosis, urolithiasis, genital infection or bladder neck obstruction was detected in SIC patients compared to the population as a whole. Vesico-ureteric reflux was noted in 9% of SIC patients compared to 6% of the population. Urethral injuries occurred in some 10% of SIC patients compared with 3.5% of patients on other forms of drainage and urinary infections occurred in 25% of SIC patients (Berard et al. 1985). However, a report of 24 female patients managed by SIC showed that almost 30% of them failed to maintain the programme for reasons of poor motivation, upper limb function or inconvenience (Joiner and Lindan 1982). In addition, although the use of anticholinergic agents may decrease reflex activity in the upper motor neurone bladder, a number of these patients will fail to be managed by SIC. The long-term bladder drainage technique of choice is SIC, with many advantages relating to the incidence of urosepsis, but other techniques may have to be employed in a proportion of patients.

Suprapubic tapping and expression of the bladder with condom drainage with or without an external sphincterotomy is an alternative long-term management technique, particularly in males with upper motor neurone lesion (Grundy and Russell 1986). Surgery to relieve bladder outlet obstruction was required in 44% of spinal cord injuries in one series and this high rate of intervention is justified by a low death rate (0.5%) from renal failure in those patients (Webb et al. 1984). The advantage regarding sepsis is the fact that the bladder does not require to be catheterised, but the wearing of condom collection systems may be associated with an increased incidence of urinary infection with kinking of the tube presumably being a major causative factor (Hirsh et al. 1979). This drainage technique is also, of course, less socially acceptable to the majority of patients.

Many patients may require chronic indwelling catheters either because of poor emptying, incontinence, poor upper limb function or an elderly or frail state (Anderson 1986; Grundy and Russell 1986). This may be a satisfactory form of drainage in selected patients but there is an increased incidence of complications and impairment of renal function (Hardy 1968; Hackler 1982). Attempts to prevent colonisation of the urinary drainage bag with bacteria have not significantly altered the incidence of infection in these patients (Burke et al. 1981). Other complications of long-term management by indwelling urethral catheters include insidious balloon deflation, occlusion of the lumen of the catheter and failure of the balloon to deflate when required (Hardy 1968).

Diagnosis of Urinary Tract Infection

The standard microbiological diagnosis of urinary tract infection is established by microscopic examination of a mid stream urine specimen combined with urinary culture and sensitivity analysis, where a significant colony count ($>10^6$ per ml) is observed. In non spinal cord injured patients on catheter drainage, these standard indices do not apply as the catheter will, in itself, induce urinary leucocytosis and a raised bacterial count. For the same reasons, diagnosis of urinary infection is difficult in spinal cord injured patients, as there is inherent urinary stasis and catheterisation is a frequent occurrence. How then may a significant urinary tract infection requiring treatment be diagnosed?

A urine testing technique is required which can rapidly and accurately detect bacteria and white cells in the urine and this test should be simple as regular testing is required. Dipstick detection of bacteria has been shown to be inaccurate (Lenke and Vandarsten 1981). A dip-slide culture technique has been advocated as a preliminary screening test, where identification of the infecting organism is only pursued if there are $>10^4$ colonies per ml of urine on two successive days (Anderson and Hatami-Tehrani 1979). A colony count of 1000 per ml with the same micro-organism in three consecutive specimens is used as a diagnostic criterion in patients on 8-hourly SIC by some workers (Pearman 1971). Other authors established the cut-off point of contamination infection as being between 10^4–10^5 bacteria per ml even for catheterised urine (Kass 1956; Reber 1967). A combination of bacteriuria ($>10^5$ per ml) and urinary leucocytosis (>20 WBC/HPF of spun urine) has also been used (Joiner and Lindan 1982). Other workers believe that any specimen of urine which contains $>10^3$ organisms is a significant infection (Rhame and Perkash 1979).

Having established what the cut-off point for significant numbers of bacteria and/or white cells is, the next problem is what constitutes an infection which requires treatment. Some workers believe that asymptomatic bateriuria is a harmless state in relation to intermittent catheterisation (Lapides et al. 1976) and the frequent detection of opportunistic organisms without evidence of impairment of function would support this theory (Lindan and Joiner 1984). However, it could be argued that the use of symptomatology as a deciding factor might be hazardous, since absence of symptoms could be due to lack of visceral sensation. The degree of pyuria associated with bacteriuria may provide evidence as to whether bacterial invasion of tissues is occurring as pyuria is, after all, the host response to infection (Anderson 1986). Antibody coating of bacteria has been suggested as a means of assessing asymptomatic bacteriuria and, although some workers believed that this is in an index of tissue invasion (Newman et al. 1980), others have not found this technique so helpful (Lindan 1981).

Localisation of infection can be important in patients with recurrent sepsis, the source of which is unknown. Differentiation between upper and lower urinary tract infection can be made using the bladder wash out test (Fairley et al. 1967; Wyndaele et al. 1983). A Foley catheter is inserted into the bladder and a specimen of urine obtained. The bladder is then emptied and neomycin solution instilled for 30 minutes. After repeated washing further specimens are obtained following injection of frusemide and the bacteria counts from the bladder and from the upper tract effluent are compared. Prostatic cystoscopic localisation of infection is a means of assessing the prostate gland as a source of recurrent urinary tract infection (Stamey 1980). Serial samples of urine from the bladder and from the prostatic urethra following prostatic massage are compared. Renal tomography may also be useful to detect renal calculi which are not seen on routine X-rays. Localisation of the source of infection based on the site of symptoms is certainly unreliable (Fairley et al. 1971).

Antimicrobial Therapy

Overview

One of the major controversial issues in the management of urinary tract infection in spinal cord injured patients is the question of whether antimicrobial prophylaxis should be used on a routine basis. It has been argued that antibiotic prophylaxis in these patients is cheaper than treatment and is a logical therapeutic principle in the neuropathic bladder, given their susceptibility to infections, calculi, reflux, hydronephrosis and chronic changes within the bladder wall (Anderson 1986).

However, other authors believe that the early use of prophylactic antibiotics is still a matter of debate (Dolfus and Gschaedler 1987). It is important that each unit establishes standard policy for antibiotic therapy, whether prophylactic or to treat established infection, and that antibiotic abuse with consequent emergence of resistant strains is prevented. It has been suggested that a microbiologist be included in the rehabilitation team and that a simple laboratory in close proximity to the spinal cord injury unit be established (Lindan 1978).

Prophylaxis

Oral

The role of antibiotic prophylaxis in spinal cord injury patients can best be assessed from the results of clinical studies where this management policy has been implemented. Low-dose antibiotic therapy (methenamine mandelate 1 g q.i.d., nitrofurantoin 50 mg b.d., or cotrimoxazole 1 tablet b.d.) was used in female patients undergoing self intermittent catheterisation and 43% of these patients were found to have significant bacteriuria on routine follow-up (Joiner and Lindan 1982). A series of 50 patients with recent spinal cord trauma who had been treated by clean intermittent catheterisation were subjected to a randomised comparison of no prophylaxis versus cotrimoxazole administered orally and although the probability of laboratory infection was significantly reduced, the likelihood of clinical infection of the urinary tract was not (Maynard and Diokno 1984). A prospective study of the efficacy of low-dose nitrofurantoin as a means of preventing urinary tract infection in spinal cord injury patients suggested that this agent is effective in preventing repeated invasion of the bladder by pathogens (Lindan and Joiner 1984). In addition the authors found this agent to be relatively non-toxic and did not cause the emergence of drug-resistant strains. They initially assessed cotrimoxazole as preventive therapy and abandoned this agent following the emergence of a drug-resistant *Enterobacter*. A comparison of cotrimoxazole, nalidixic acid, methenamine hippurate, nitrofurantoin macrocrystals, ascorbic acid or no prophylaxis was made in 151 male patients (Kuhlemeier et al. 1985). None of these agents was effective in reducing the incidence of bacteriuria in these patients and organisms emerged with resistance to a number of these drugs. The authors concluded that oral prophylaxis was not indicated in patients on inter-mittent catheterisation (Kuhlemeier et al. 1985).

In this study ascorbic acid was particularly ineffective. Cotrimoxazole has been assessed in another study and found to be no better than no treatment in preven-ting urinary tract infection (Thorsteinsson and Kees 1983), but other workers have produced contradictory evidence (Merritt et al. 1982). In other studies, nitrofuran-toin, methenamine salts in conjunction with hemiacidrin, methenamine salts and ascorbic acid, and methenamine mandelate with ammonium chloride have all been of benefit in reducing bacteriuria in spinal cord injury patients to a greater or lesser degree (Anderson 1980; Krebs et al. 1984; Merritt et al. 1982; Kevorkian 1984).

The results from these studies clearly show the controversy that exists regar-ding oral prophylaxis and this is in contrast to results obtained from oral prophylaxis in patients with normal bladder function who have recurrent urinary tract infections, where treatment has been clearly of benefit (Stamey 1980). There is no doubt that the chronic use of prophylactic antibiotics is associated with the risk of emergence of highly resistant and virulent organisms and this argument has been made and supported by data showing that no treatment or prophylaxis is required for chronic bacteriuria in spinal cord injured patients (Lewis et al. 1984).

Intravesical

Regarding prophylaxis with bladder irrigants, routine use following intermittent catheterisation might seem a logical and appropriate therapy, as this would eradicate inoculated organisms (Anderson 1986). In fact, results of irrigant prophylaxis have been more encouraging than those where oral agents were used. A combination of kanamycin and colistin instilled following intermittent catheterisation has been associated with a low incidence of bacteriuria (Pearman 1971). Likewise, other workers have found benefit from a combination of neomycin and polymyxin B (Rhame and Perkash 1979).

A comparison was made between three antiseptic agents (phenoxyethanol, chlorhexidine and noxythiolin) in patients with indwelling catheters (Stickler et al. 1981a). In this study, phenoxyethanol was effective against all common urinary pathogens tested and chlorhexidine was effective against most organisms with the exception of *Providencia stuartii*. Noxythiolin had little effect on any of the pathogens and this was thought to be due to inadequate decomposition of this substance to produce formaldehyde in the presence of abnormal urine constituents. Phenoxyethanol was therefore concluded to be an effective agent for use as a prophylactic bladder irrigant. When 57 Gram-negative bacterial isolates from urinary tract infections in spinal cord injury patients were tested for sensitivity to chlorhexidine, cetrimide, glutaraldehyde and a proprietary antiseptic (Resiguard), a substantial percentage were resistant to chlorhexidine, cetrimide and Resiguard. The species which were resistant to the antiseptics were also resistant to a range of antibiotics. From this study it was concluded that the extensive use of such antiseptic agents might lead to selection of highly drug-resistant organisms (Stickler et al. 1981b). It was advised that if antiseptic agents are to be used as irrigants in the bladder, they should be ones which are negatively correlated with drug sensitivity. One further irrigant of interest is Suby-G solution, which contains citric acid 3.23% and can be of benefit in preventing stone encrustation on the balloon of an indwelling catheter (Grundy et al. 1986).

Other Methods

Regarding other methods of prophylaxis, it has been suggested that where indwelling catheters are used with a 100% infection rate, the best prophylaxis is a high fluid intake to maintain an adequate through-put of urine and minimise colonisation (O'Flynn 1974). In addition acetohydroxamic acid, which is a urease inhibitor, may help prevent growth of infected renal calculi (Griffith et al. 1978).

Summarising the data from studies of various forms of prophylaxis, it appears that antibiotic or antiseptic preventive therapy is associated with a significant risk of colonisation with resistant organisms. In this regard, a high fluid intake can be recommended as an effective and safe form of prophylaxis.

Treatment of Infection

The principles of treatment of acute infective episodes are similar in spinal cord injured patients to those in the general population. The infecting organism must be accurately identified, the urinary tract adequately drained, flow of urine promoted and the appropriate antibiotic administered, if necessary systemically. If a patient is on intermittent catheterisation, it may be prudent to temporarily establish continuous drainage which will allow free intake of fluids without necessitating frequent intermittent catheterisations. In addition there is the risk that organisms can multiply within the bladder in the period between catheterisations (Silver 1974).

Where there is infection with resistant organisms such as *Providencia*, it is advisable to discontinue all antibiotics and allow time to elapse for the bladder to be colonised by a less resistant organism (Silver 1974). It must be emphasised that *Pseudomonas* may in many cases be a harmless and even symbiotic commensal (Lindan and Joiner 1984) but, where therapy is indicated for

Pseudomonas infection with systemic manifestations, cefsulodin is recommended for treatment of this organism as it has been shown to be much more effective than aminoglycosides (Montgomerie et al. 1986). The advantage of this agent is that it has a narrow spectrum and will not select resistant bacteria, resulting in superinfection.

The reservation of antibiotics for infective episodes with systemic manifestations is recommended as a baseline policy, with exceptions where the urine is colonised by a single organism with a markedly high colony count or for persistent colonisation by *Proteus* which is associated with the highest incidence of calculi (Grundy and Russell 1986). Asymptomatic bacteriuria should not routinely be treated by antibiotic therapy in spinal cord injured patients.

Surgery

Operative surgical procedures may be indicated in some cases where urinary tract infections in spinal cord injured patients are persistent and problematic. When investigation reveals that unilateral renal pathology is the source for recurring infection, there are two circumstances where nephro-ureterectomy may be indicated. First the presence of pyonephrosis in a kidney which is poorly functioning may best be treated by nephrectomy. In addition if a kidney has been shown to be the source of recurrent infection by individual ureteric urine sampling and is also known to be a poorly functioning unit, a nephrectomy may again be a reasonable option. Vesico-ureteric reflux may, in the presence of chronic cystitis, give rise to recurring ascending pyelonephritis. The establishment of adequate bladder drainage and the use of antibiotics may cause reversal of this condition provided the bladder wall has not been damaged beyond repair (Ross et al. 1960). If these measures fail to correct vesico-ureteric reflux, antireflux surgery may be indicated (Gibbon 1974). Finally, surgical removal of calculi may be required in spinal cord injury patients, particularly when associated sepsis is resistant to antibiotic therapy alone. Cystoscopic litholapaxy is used to remove bladder calculi. In recent years, the application of percutaneous nephrolithotomy, ureteroscopy and extracorporeal shock wave lithotripsy have been major advances in the ability to treat calculous disease. These procedures enable treatment of sepsis related to renal and ureteric calculi without the morbidity and scarring associated with open renal or ureteric surgery. However, surgical procedures for calculous disease are uncommon in spinal cord injured patients according to one series (Webb et al. 1984).

Future Prospects

The introduction of urodynamic evaluation has led to major advances in diagnostic accuracy in spinal cord injured patients and self intermittent catheterisation has given rise to a greatly improved quality of life. There are at least two prospects under present evaluation which may be further advances in management. Sacral anterior root stimulators may provide a means for improving control of bladder function (Brindley et al. 1982) although their role in the management of spinal cord injured patients has yet to be established. In addition, the use of artificial sphincters, which has been a routine practice for the treatment of selected incontinence patients, may have a significant role in some patients whose bladder is acontractile and incontinent. Such procedures may reduce the need for catheterisation techniques and result in improvement in the rate of urosepsis. Finally, the advent and application of computer data storage systems can be developed to allow useful and accurate comparison of treatments and results within and between spinal cord trauma units.

Summary

Adequate bladder drainage was the first step towards improved mortality and morbidity in spinal cord injured patients. Intermittent catheterisation while in hospital, followed by self intermittent catheterisation, has provided a simple, cheap and acceptable means of achieving this end and should be applied to patients with a neuropathic bladder whenever possible. The advent of potent and specific pharmacological agents which can reduce activity within the neuropathic bladder has greatly enhanced the application of this technique.

Regarding antimicrobial therapy, it must always be remembered that the equilibrium between host and pathogen always depends on a third factor: suppression of pathogen by competition with co-existing commensal organisms. Therefore, it is imprudent to attempt prevention of colonisation of the urinary tract in spinal cord injured patients by chronic suppression of pathogenic organisms. The recommended policy is to maintain host pathogen equilibrium by ensuring the general well being of the patient, adequate drainage of the urinary tract and preservation of a healthy bacterial commensal environment. Antimicrobial therapy should be reserved for accurate and effective use during episodes of significant clinical infection.

References

Anderson RU (1980) Prophylaxis of bacteriuria during intermittent catheterisation of the acute neurogenic bladder. J Urol 123: 364

Anderson RU (1986) Urinary tract infections in spinal cord injury patients. In: Walsh PC, Gittes RF, Perlmutter AD, Stemi TA (eds) Campbell's Urology. Saunders, Philadelphia, pp 888–898

Anderson RU, Hatami-Tehrani G (1979) Monitoring for bacteriuria in spinal cord injured patients on intermittent catheterization. Urology 14: 244–248

Ascoli R (1968) The indwelling catheter in paraplegics with particular reference to urethral diverticula. Paraplegia 6: 17–21

Barton CH, Vaziri ND, Gordon S, Tilles S (1984) Renal pathology in end stage renal disease associated with paraplegia. Paraplegia 22: 31–41

Berard E, Depassio J, Pangaod N, Landi J (1985) Self catheterisation; urinary complications and the social resettlement of spinal cord injured patients. Paraplegia 32: 386–388

Bouchard C (1989) Influence qu'exercice sur la maladie charbonneuse l'inoculation du bacille pyocycanique. C R Seances Acad Sci (Paris) 108: 713–714

Bradley WE, Chou S, French LA (1963) Further experience with a radiotransmitter receiver unit for the neurogenic bladder. J Neurosurg 20: 953–960

Bradley WE, Chou S, Markland C (1967) In: Boyarski S (ed) The neurogenic bladder. Williams and Wilkins, Baltimore, pp 139–145

Brindley GS, Polkey CE, Rushton DM (1982) Sacral anterior root stimulators for bladder control in paraplegia. Paraplegia 20: 365–381

Burke JP, Garibali RA, Britt MR, Jacobson JA, Conti M (1981) Prevention of catheter associated urinary tract infection. Am J Med 70: 655–660

Cardenas DD, Mayo M (1987) Bacteriuria with fever after spinal cord injury. Arch Phys Med Rehabil 68: 291–293

Comarr AE (1961) Chronic infection of the urinary tract among patients with spinal cord injury. J Urol 85: 9–13

Comarr AE, Kawaichi GK, Bors E (1962) Renal calculosis of patients with traumatic cord lesion. J Urol 87: 647–656

Cooke JB, Smith PH (1968) Long term urethral catheterisation after spinal injury. Paraplegia 6: 11–16

De Vivo MJ, Fine P, Cutter GR, Maetz HM (1984) The risk of renal calculi in spinal cord injury patients. J Urol 131: 857–860

Dollfus P, Gschaedler R (1987) Initial hospital care of spinal cord injury patients. Paraplegia 25: 241–243

Fairley FK, Bond AG, Brown RB Harbersberger P (1967) Simple test to determine the site of urinary tract infection. Lancet 2: 427–428

Fairley FK, Carson NE, Gutch RS (1971) Site of infection in acute urinary tract infection in general practice. Lancet 2: 615–618

Gardner BP, Parsons KF, Machin DG, Galloway A, Krishnan R (1986) The urological management of spinal cord damaged patients: a clinical algorithm. Paraplegia 24: 138–147

Gibbon NOK (1966) Management of the bladder in acute and chronic disorders of the nervous system. Acta Urol Scand (Suppl) 42: 133–136

Gibbon NOK (1974) Later management of the paraplegic bladder. Paraplegia 12: 87–91

Gilmore DS, Shick DG, Montgomerie JZ (1982) *Pseudomonas aeruginosa* colonization in patients with spinal cord injuries. J Clin Microbiol 16: 865–867

Glahn BE (1970) Manual of provocation of micturition contraction in neurogenic bladder. Scand J Urol Nephrol 4: 25–30

Golden JSR (1968) Early management of traumatic paraplegia in males. Rehabilitation 66: 49–54

Grainger R, O'Flynn JD, Fitzpatrick JM (1988) Urological follow-up of 107 females following spinal cord injury. J Urol (Suppl) 139: 512A

Griffith HM, Gibson JR, Clinton CW, Musher DM (1978) Acetohydroxamic acid: clinical studies of a urease inhibitor in patients with staghorn renal calculi. J Urol 119: 9–15

Gross GW, Liebowitz RL (1981) Infection does not cause reflux. Am J Radiol 137: 929–932

Grundy D, Russell J (1986) ABC of spinal cord injury: urological management. Br Med J 292: 249–253

Grundy DJ, Fellows GJ, Gillett AP, Nuseibeh I, Silver JR (1983) A comparison of fine bore suprapubic and an intermittent urethral catheterisation regime after spinal cord injury. Paraplegia 21: 227–232

Grundy D, Swaine A, Russell J (1986) ABC of spinal cord injury: early management and complications II. Br Med J 292: 123–125

Guttman L (1976) Spinal cord injuries: comprehensive management and research. Blackwell, Oxford

Guttman L, Frankel H (1966) The value of intermittent catheterisation in the early management of traumatic paraplegia and tetraplegia. Paraplegia 4: 63–83

Hackler RH (1982) Long term suprapubic cystostomy drainage in spinal cord injury patients. Br J Urol 54: 120–121

Hardy AG (1968) Complications of the indwelling urethral catheter. Int J Paraplegia 6: 5–7

Hirsh DD, Fainstein V, Musher DM (1979) Do condom catheter collection systems cause urinary tract infection? JAMA 242: 340–342

Jameson RM (1969) Surgical management of the neurogenic bladder and its complications. Br J Clin Pract 23: 359–363

Joiner E, Lindan R (1982) Experience with self intermittent catheterisation for women with neurological dysfunctions of the bladder. Paraplegia 20: 147–153

Kass EA (1956) Asymptomatic infections of the urinary tract. Trans Assoc Am Physicians 69: 56–59

Kass EJ, Koff SA, Diokno AC, Lapides J (1981) The significance of bacilluria in children on long term intermittent catheterisation. J Urol 126: 223–227

Kevorkian CG., Merritt JL, Ilstrup DM (1984) Methenamine mandelate with acidification: an effective urinary antiseptic in patients with neurogenic bladder. Mayo Clin Proc 59: 523–528

Kohli A, Lamid S (1986) Risk factors for renal stone formation in patients with spinal cord injury. Br J Urol 58: 588–591

Krebs M, Halvorsen RB, Fishman IJ, Santos-Mendoza N (1984) Prevention of urinary tract infection during catheterisation. J Urol 131: 82–86

Kuhlemeier KV, Stover SL, Lloyd LK (1985) Prophylactic antibacterial therapy for preventing urinary tract infections in spinal cord injury patients. J Urol 134: 514–517

Kyle EQ (1968) The complications of indwelling catheters. Paraplegia 6: 1–4

Lapides J (1973) Pathophysiology of urinary tract infections. University of Michigan Medical Center Journal 39: 103–106

Lapides J, Diokno AC, Silver SJ, Lower BS (1972) Clean intermittent catheterisation in the treatment of urinary tract disease. J Urol 107: 458–461

Lapides J, Diokno AC, Gould FR, Lowe BS (1976) Further observations on self catheterisation. J Urol 116: 169–172

Lenke RR, Vandarsten JP (1981) The efficacy of the nitrite test and microscopic analysis in predicting urine culture results. Am J Obstet Gynecol 140: 427–429

Lewis RI, Carrion HM, Lockhart JL Politano VA (1984) Significance of asymptomatic bacteriuria in neurogenic bladder disease. Urology 23: 343–345

Lindan R (1978) The role of the microbiologist in the treatment and rehabilitation of patients with spinal cord injuries. Paraplegia 16: 237–241

Lindan R (1981) The significance of antibody coated bacteria in uropathic bladder urines. Paraplegia 19: 216–222

Lindan R, Joiner E (1984) A prospective study of the efficacy of low dose nitrofurantoin in preventing urinary tract infections in spinal cord injury patients, with comments on the role of pseudomonads. Paraplegia 22: 61–65

Lloyd-Davies RW, Hinman F Jr (1971) Structural and functional changes leading to impaired bacteria elimination after overdistension of the rabbit bladder. Invest Urol 9: 136–139

Lloyd-Davies RW, Clarke AE, Prout WG, Shuttleworth KED, Tighe JR (1970) The effects of stretching the rabbit bladder. Preliminary observations. Invest Urol 8: 145–147

Maynard FM, Diokno AC (1984) Urinary infection and complications during clean intermittent catheterisation following spinal cord injury. J Urol 132: 943–946

Merritt JL (1981) Residual urine volume: correlate of urinary tract infection in patients with spinal cord injury. Arch Phys Med Rehabil. 62: 558–561

Merritt JL, Ericson RP, Optiz JL, (1982) Bacteriuria during follow up in patients with spinal cord injury: efficacy of antimicrobial suppressants. Arch Phys Med Rehabil 63: 413–416

Miller JM (1971) Bacteriuria in 50 patients now catheter free after a period of long term Foley catheter drainage. In: Proceedings of 18th Veterans' Administration, Spinal Cord injury Conference Harvard Medical School, Boston, pp 148–154

Montgomerie JA, Morrow JW (1980) Long term pseudomonas colonization in spinal cord injury patients. Am J Epidemiol 112: 508–512

Montgomerie JA, Morrow, JW, Canawait HN, Gilmore DS, Graham IE, Ibraham MZ (1986) Cefsulodin in treatment of pseudomonas urinary tract infection in patients with spinal cord injury. Urology 28: 446–450

Newman E, Price M, Ederer GM (1980) Urinary tract infection in patients with spinal cord lesions: antibody coated bacteria test as a diagnostic aid. Arch Phys Med Rehabil 61: 406–409

Nikakhtar B, Paziri N, Khansari F, Gordon S, Mirahmadi M (1981) Urolithisis in patients with spinal cord injury. Paraplegia 19: 363–366

O'Flynn JD (1974) Early management of neuropathic bladder in spinal cord injuries. Paraplegia 12: 83–86

O'Grady F, Cattell WR (1966) Kinetics of urinary tract infection. II The bladder. Br J Urol 38: 156–162

Optiz J (1984) Treatment of voiding dysfunction in spinal cord injured patients; bladder retaining. In: Barrett D, Wein A (eds) Controversies in neuroneurology. Churchill Livingstone, New York pp 437–451

Ott R, Rossier AB (1971) The importance of intermittent catheterisation in bladder re-education of acute traumatic spinal cord lesions. In: Proceedings of the 18th Veterans' Administration, Spinal Cord Injury Conference, Harvard Medical Center, Boston, pp 139–148

Pearman JW (1971) Prevention of urinary tract infection following spinal cord injury. Paraplegia 9: 95–105

Pearman JW (1976) Urological follow up of 99 spinal cord injured patients initially managed by intermittent catheterisation. Br J Urol 48: 297–310

Pearman JW, England EJ (1973) The urological management of the patient following spinal cord injury. Thomas, Springfield, Illinois

Peatfield RC, Burt AA, Smith PH (1983) Suprapubic catheterisation after spinal cord injury: a follow-up report. Paraplegia 21: 220–226

Perkash I (1974) Intermittent catheterisation: the urologist's point of view. J Urol 111: 356–360

Reber H (1967) Zur Diagnose des Harnwegsinfektes Praxis 56: 779–782

Rhame FS, Perkash I (1979) Urinary tract infection occurring in recent spinal cord injury patients on intermittent catherization. J Urol 122: 669–672

Ross JC, Damanski M, Gibbon N (1960) Ureteric reflux in the paraplegic. Br J Surg 47: 536–642

Rossier AB, Bushra AF (1979) From intermittent catheterisation to catheter freedom via urodynamics: a tribute to Sir Ludwig Guttman. Paraplegia 17: 73–85

Sharpe JR, Comarr AE, Fuelleman R (1971) Long term catheter drainage in the neurogenic bladder. In: Proceedings of the 18th Veterans' Administration Spinal Cord Injury Conference, Harvard Medical School, Boston, pp 125–132

Silver JR (1974) Management of urinary tract infection in acute paraplegic patients with special reference to the paper strip screening test for infection. Paraplegia 12: 50–60

Smith PH, Cook JB, Rhine JR (1972) Manual expression of the bladder following spinal injury. Paraplegia 9: 213–218

Stamey TA (1980) Pathogenesis and treatment of urinary tract infections. Williams and Wilkins, Baltimore, pp 555–562

Stickler DJ, Wilmot CB, O'Flynn JD (1970) The mode of development of urinary infection in intermittently catheterised male paraplegics. Int J Paraplegia 8: 243–245

Stickler DJ, Plant S, Bunni NH, Chawla JC (1981a) Some observations on the activity of three antiseptics used as bladder irrigants in the treatment of urinary tract infection in patients with indwelling catheters. Paraplegia 19: 325–333

Stickler DJ Thomas B, Chawla JC (1981b) Antiseptic and antibiotic resistance in gram-negative bacteria causing urinary tract infection in spinal cord injury patients. Paraplegia 19: 50–56

Thompson-Walker JW (1917) The bladder in gunshot and other injuries of the spinal cord. Lancet 1: 173–179

Thorsteinsson G, Kees T (1983) The frequency and type of urinary tract infections in patients on intermittent catheterisation by self and by catheterisation team. Arch Phys Med Rehabil 4: 519–523

Vargus A, Bragin S, Mendez R (1982) Staghorn calculus: its clinical presentation, complications and management. J Urol 127: 860–862

Walsh JJ (1968) Further experience with intermittent catheterisation. Paraplegia 6: 74–79

Webb DR, Fitzpatrick JM, O'Flynn JD (1984) A 15-year follow-up of 406 consecutive spinal cord injuries. Br J Urol 56: 614–617

Wein A (1984) Pharmacology of the bladder and urethra. In: Mundy A, Stephenson T, Wein A (eds) Urodynamics. Churchill Livingstone, Edinburgh, pp 26–41

Wyndaele JJ, Oosterlinck W, DeSy WA, Claessens H (1983) The use of the bladder wash out test in patients with spinal cord lesions who have urinary tract infection. Paraplegia 21: 294–300

Wyndaele J, DeSy WA, Claessens N (1985) Evaluation of different methods of bladder drainage used in the early care of spinal cord injury patients. Paraplegia 23: 18–26

Wyndaele JJ (1987) Urology in spinal cord injured patients. Paraplegia 25: 267–269

Young JS (1982) Spinal cord injury statistics: experience of regional spinal injury systems. Good Samaritan Medical Center, Phoenix, pp 34–35

Chapter 7

Sexual and Fertility Concerns

Surgical Considerations

D.A. Ohl and C.J. Bennett

Introduction

Society tends to think of the disabled person as asexual (Cole 1975a). This is not true. The majority of spinal cord injured (SCI) patients are young and they tend to have young partners. Because of this, sexuality and fertility potential are of great concern. In this chapter we will review the sexual and fertility capabilities of the SCI patient and discuss techniques which may be used to improve them.

Physiology of Erection and Ejaculation

Erection

The blood flow to the penis is derived from the internal pudendal artery, which gives rise to the dorsal, the cavernosal and the spongiosal arteries. The erectile bodies are supplied by the cavernosal arteries, and there is free communication of blood between them. The dorsal artery supplies the penile skin and glans penis, while the spongiosal artery supplies the corpus spongiosum.

There are three major subdivisions to the venous drainage of the penis (Newman and Northrup 1981). The skin and prepuce are drained by the superficial dorsal vein which usually terminates in the saphenous vein. The intermediate system consists of the deep dorsal vein and feeding vessels from the glans. The deep dorsal veins receive blood from the cavernous bodies via the emissary veins which pierce the tunica albuginea along its length. The deep system includes veins of the corpus spongiosum and the deep veins of the penis which exit from the proximal corpus cavernosum.

During erection, the arterial inflow to the penis increases markedly (Karacan et al. 1983) and blood is selectively shunted to the cavernous spaces of the corporal bodies (Krane and Siroky 1981). Most investigators feel this is primarily an arterial event. Conti (1952) theorised that opening or closing of Ebner's cushions caused increased flow to the cavernous bodies while decreasing venous outflow during erection. In the flaccid state, these polsters would open arteriovenous shunts and venous channels to allow bypass of the corporal bodies. The universal existence of polsters and their role in controlling erection, however, is not universally accepted (Benson et al. 1981).

The vascular changes of erection are under complex neurological control. The major motor supply to the penis is the sacral parasympathetic nerves. Eckhardt (1863) demonstrated that electrical stimulation of these nerves produced erection in dogs. It was subsequently shown by ganglionic blockade that these parasympathetic nerves are preganglionic and that intra-arterial injection of acetylcholine did not cause erection (Dorr and Brody 1967). Other studies have suggested that the final neutotransmitter may be adrenergic (Domer et al. 1978; Siroky and Krane 1983) or that it may be vasoactive intestinal polypeptide (Ottesen et al. 1983).

Psychogenic mediated erection can occur via thoracolumbar sympathetic nerves as demonstrated experimentally in the cat (Root and Bard 1947) and clinically in complete sacral cord-injured man (Bors and Comarr 1960). This pathway certainly is not necessary for erection as sympathectomy from retroperitoneal lymph node dissection does not result in impotence (Kedia et al. 1975).

The sensory supply to the penis is carried by the dorsal nerves of the penis and the internal pudendal nerves which enter the spinal cord at S2–4. This pathway and the sacral parasympathetic outflow create the arc responsible for reflexogenic erections.

Ejaculation

Ejaculation is a complex process, which may be caused by reflex genital stimulation or by cortical input. The afferent input into the ejaculatory reflex is via the dorsal nerves of the penis. Efferent fibres are the sympathetics arising from T11–L2, which exit the sympathetic chain to form the hypogastric plexus before coursing into the pelvis to join the parasympathetic nerves. Synapses with short adrenergic neurones are located on the surface of the bladder neck, vas deferens, seminal vesicles, epididymis, and prostate (Thomas 1983).

Contraction of the vas deferens propels spermatozoa to the ampulla, and contraction of the prostate, seminal vesicles and ampulla creates emission of seminal fluid into the posterior urethra. Emission and simultaneous bladder neck closure (which prevents retrograde ejaculation) are under sympathetic control. Projectile ejaculation of the fluid by pelvic musculature is effected through sacral parasympathetics (Kedia 1983).

Baseline Sexual Capability of SCI Patients

Erection and Ejaculation

Table 7.1 is a compilation of data from several large studies on sexual capabilities of SCI males. This is not a complete list of papers written on the subject, but most of the large studies on the topic are included.

Munro et al. (1948) studied 84 men with spinal cord injuries of varying aetiology. In this study, the degree of completeness of the injury had no bearing on the frequency of erection or ejaculation. An intact sacral cord, as judged by anal reflex and bladder function, was associated with a higher incidence of erections but it was not a requirement. Extensive damage to the cord between T8 and L3 was associated with absence of ejaculation. Two patients in the series successfully impregnated their wives; one, a complete T6 paraplegic and the other an incomplete C5 quadriplegic.

Talbot (1955) surveyed 408 US veterans on their sexual capabilities after spinal cord injury. Sixty-six per cent of all patients had erectile capability with approximately one-third achieving erection psychogenically and two-thirds by reflex. Talbot theorised that psychogenic erections were possible because of incompleteness of the lesion. There was a much higher incidence of ejaculation (44%) in patients with psychogenic erections. The observation was made that lumbosacral injuries had a lower incidence of erection. It was estimated that 5% of these men were fertile.

Zeitlin et al. (1957) found a correlation between higher spinal level and ability to have erections. All of their patients had "ample opportunity" out of the hospital to attempt intercourse. Thirty-eight attempted intercourse and 26 were successful. Only three had external ejaculation and only one pregnancy was seen, despite a total of 88 pregnancies among the group prior to injury.

Bors and Comarr (1960) divided their 529 patients into upper motor neurone/lower motor neurone and complete/incomplete lesions. Erection was more common in upper motor neurone lesions, while ejaculation was more common with lower motor neurone lesions. They pointed out the importance of the lower thoracic/upper lumbar outflow in causing psychogenic erections in complete lower motor neurone lesions (27%).

Tsuji et al. (1961) also showed that the higher complete lesion group had more erectile capability but noted that the level of lesion had less impact if the lesion

Table 7.1 Data compiled from several studies on the sexual capabilities of spinal cord injured males

Reference	n	Erection		Ejaculation		
		No.	%	No.	%	Fertile
Munro et al. (1948)	84	62	74	7	8	3 (3%)
Talbot (1955)	408	270	66	55	13	est 5%
Zeitlin et al. (1957)	100	64	64	3	3	1(1%)
Bors and Comarr (1960)	529	427	80	80	15	18 (3%)
Tsuji et al. (1961)	638	341	54	60	9	0
Comarr (1970)	150	123	82	16	11	0

was incomplete. Again, lower lesions tended to have a higher incidence of ejaculation in both the complete and incomplete groups. Coitus was attempted in 53 and was successful in 32 (60% of those attempting).

In summary, erection is noted to occur in 54%–82% of SCI males. Ejaculation occurs in 3%–15%. The return of sexual function coincides with emergence from spinal shock. Erection is more common in upper motor neurone lesions, higher level lesions and incomplete lesions. Ejaculation is more common in lesions that are lower motor neurone, lower in the cord, and incomplete. The incidence of fertility in these studies was 0%–5%. Lower and incomplete lesions were more fertile. Comarr (1970) corroborates these findings, but notes that individual variation prevents using the lesion characteristics to predict accurately the individual patient's sexual potential. We agree with this, and never speak in *definite* terms regarding future sexual prospects early after injury.

Testicular Function

There are several reports that spermatogenesis is impaired in spinal cord injured males. Bors et al. (1950) found abnormalities in all but 3 of 35 testicular biopsy specimens and Tsuji et al. (1961) found abnormalities in 70%. On the other hand, Perkash et al. (1985) found normal or only mildly reduced spermatogenesis in 12 of 13 paraplegics. Talbot (1971) stated that the incidence of testicular atrophy is decreasing.

Whether hormonal changes cause impaired spermatogenesis is controversial. Bors et al. (1950) noted decreased urinary gonadotrophins and increased urinary oestrogens and 17-ketosteroids, but did not comment on the significance. More recently, elevated follicle-stimulating hormone (FSH) and luteinising hormone (LH) levels have been identified with normal testosterone and prolactin levels (Hayes et al. 1979). Other studies have not identified these endocrine abnormalities (Kikuchi et al. 1976; David et al. 1977) or have had mixed results (Morley et al. 1979).

Evidence for a "neurogenic testicle" was argued by Bors et al. (1950) and Leriche et al. (1977). They cite the fact that lower level and/or incomplete lesions which preserve testicular sensation are associated with less impairment of spermatogenesis. One wonders, however, if this association simply reflects the idea that intact sensation causes avoidance of painful external stimuli, which might be damaging to the testis or directs the patient to treatment of epididymitis at an earlier stage than higher level lesions. We tell patients to make an active attempt to avoid testicular trauma in daily activity.

Scrotal hyperthemia has been suggested as a cause for poor spermatogenesis in paraplegics. Morales and Hardin (1958) found no difference in scrotal temperatures of paraplegics and controls, but more recently, Brindley (1982) measured scrotal temperature in paraplegics and found it to be 0.9°C higher than controls. A suggestion was made to prop the legs apart while sitting and to wear "scrotal-slit" underwear to keep the temperature lower.

Infection may be a cause of subfertility in SCI males. Perkash et al. (1985) felt this may be due to both direct effects of infection and also sperm-toxic medication given to treat infection, such as mandelamine. Epididymitis, a not infrequent occurrence in SCI males, may cause obstructive azoospermia (Wagenknecht 1985). Infection can also cause testicular parenchymal atrophy (Nilsson et al. 1968). It would seem that prompt treatment and/or prevention of infection should be a goal to maximise preservation of fertility.

Sexual Behaviour Patterns

There is a paucity of information regarding actual sexual practice of SCI patients. One problem in reporting is that many of the patients in large studies were hospital-bound during the surveys. Also, most large series concentrate only on the frequency of penile-vaginal intercourse. In those studies, the incidence of successful coitus in those attempting is 60%–85% (Zeitlin et al. 1957; Tsuiji et al. 1961; Comarr 1971).

Fifty male paraplegics were interviewed by Phelps et al. (1983) about their sexual techniques. Eighty-four per cent had attempted coitus with 54% succeeding. The most common sexual activities noted were oral/vaginal stimulation (78%) and stroking of the penis (76%). The technique most commonly used for achieving erection after injury was penile manipulation as opposed to the non-genital foreplay used prior to injury. The two most common reasons for decreased sexual activity were lack of opportunities (66%) and lack of personal satisfaction (59%). Of those interviewed, 42% were dissatisfied with their sex lives, and quadriplegics felt more sexually inadequate than paraplegics (83% vs 57%).

Halstead et al. (1978) interviewed 98 disabled (75% SCI patients) and 552 able-bodied people to investigate differences in sexual behaviour. The disabled group reported a lower frequency of recent masturbation (87% vs 59%), penile-vaginal intercourse (90% vs 62%) and oral-genital activity (82% vs 59%). Lack of a partner was the most common reason for decreased activity in both groups, but not being "sexually desirable" and physical problems were important reasons for avoiding sex in the disabled group, but not in the able-bodied group.

Difficulties with sexual activity may be part of the reason for avoidance. Autonomic hyperreflexia may occur with sexual stimulation in patients with high lesions. Indwelling catheters, if present, require special management. The possibility of urinary and faecal incontinence is also present.

Social Aspects

Psychological Effects

Weinberg (1982) identified five problem areas that the new SCI patient must confront before enjoying sex once again. He must accept the new body image as his own and recognise its capabilities and limitations. Along with this acceptance comes regeneration of self-esteem and worth. He must overcome the loss of gender identity, i.e. realise that he may require a great deal of assistance, yet maintain his maleness. He must be able to make new decisions regarding sexuality and parenting with the new circumstances. Finally, he must accept that the sexual experience may be entirely different than that of an able-bodied person.

Effect on Marriage

There have been conflicting reports of the effect of spinal cord injury on previous or future marriage success. Grynbaum et al. (1963) followed 47 patients. At the time of injury, 65% of males were married but after two years the percentage dropped to 33%. In contrast, the percentage of married females rose from 48% to 77%. This suggests that male SCI patients have more difficulty maintaining a marriage than females. In contrast, Guttman (1964) found that the divorce rate in his series of 975 married patients was 57/975 – somewhat greater than that of able-bodied people in the United Kingdom, but certainly the vast majority of his patients remained married despite the injury. Deyoe (1972) found a post-injury separation rate below the national average in the United States.

Sexual and Fertility Concerns of the Female SCI Patient

Sexual Experience

More women are capable of sexual intercourse following spinal cord injury than men due to lack of need of an active process, such as erection. There may, however, be differences in vaginal lubrication and swelling or contraction of the vagina and uterus depending on the level of injury (Anderson and Cole 1975). Bors and Comarr (1960) felt that vascular engorgement of the clitoris, labia and vagina, Bartholin's gland secretion, and vaginal lubrication were under the control of the S2–4 parasympathetic reflex arc.

Physiological orgasm, as in males, originates in the thoracolumbar sympathetics, and causes contraction of the uterus, uterine tubes and glands of Skene. This is followed by pelvic floor contraction mediated by S2–4. Few women with complete lesions experience orgasm (Jackson 1972).

As in males, women may experience autonomic dysreflexia during intercourse. Bladder and bowel incontinence may occur. Spasticity in a woman may make intercourse difficult due to position.

Fertility and Contraception

In 50% of cases, spinal cord injury causes transient amenorrhoea (Comarr 1966). The normal menstrual cycle usually returns within six months. Fertility is generally unimpaired.

There are various methods of contraception available to SCI women (Weinberg 1982). Condom use with spermicidal foam is an effective method which does not pose a danger to the SCI women. Likewise, a diaphragm poses no threat but there may be a problem with the patient properly positioning the device. Intrauterine devices (IUD) can be inserted without pain, but this lack of sensation may delay diagnosis and therapy of an IUD-associated pelvic inflammatory disease. Oral contraceptives should not be used in spinal cord patients because of the risk of thrombophlebitis. Again, lack of sensation may worsen the course of a thrombosis due to delay in diagnosis and the immobility of a patient may predispose her to this condition.

Pregnancy and Delivery

Although SCI women can successfully carry and deliver babies with high success, they require extra care during pregnancy. The incidence of urinary tract infection during pregnancy in these patients is high (Young et al. 1983) and fetal wastage secondary to urosepsis has been documented (Robertson 1972). Pregnancy can cause or exacerbate urinary incontinence due to increased pressure on the bladder. Anaemia, hypoproteinaemia and respiratory compromise have been noted in these patients (Ohry et al. 1978).

One study showed a somewhat higher stillbirth rate in injured patients as compared to the general population (Robertson 1972). Another showed no increase in fetal malformations in women who conceived after injury, but an increase in anomalies was seen in women injured during pregnancy (Goller and Paeslack 1972), probably as a result of the maternal trauma.

The pain afferents from the uterus are carried by thoracolumbar sympathetics. Thus, a patient with her spinal level above T10 may not appreciate the onset of labour (Robertson 1972). Unsupervised delivery may therefore ensue. This can be avoided by frequent antenatal examinations and admission to the hospital at first sign of cervical dilatation.

A patient with a high spinal lesion is at risk for autonomic dysreflexia during labour from cervical distension (Greenspoon 1986). Profound increase in blood pressure can occur and cerebrovascular accidents have been reported (Guttman et al. 1965). Epidural anaesthesia to block this dangerous reflex may be the treatment of choice (Spielman 1984; Catanzarite et al. 1984). If an anaesthetic is not used, one must be quite prepared to control very rapid changes in blood pressure with medication.

Specific Treatments of Sexual Problems

Counselling

Much of the problem with effective sexual counselling of SCI patients relates to avoidance of the topic. This may be from a variety of reasons such as lack of knowledge and anxiety in team members (Cole 1975b). The knowledge of sexuality of SCI patients was tested in a group of 30 physical therapists (Conine et al. 1979). Twenty-eight of the 40 items were answered incorrectly by at least 10% of the group. The lack of counselling by rehabilitation personnel, despite their seeing the need for it, was pointed out by Cole and Stevens (1975).

One type of attempt to correct these problems in both professionals and SCI adults has been the formation of workshops that deal with the sexual issues. A programme at the University of Minnesota (Cole et al. 1973) began with desensitisation of the participants to sexual issues. Explicit films, showing nudity, intercourse, masturbation, homosexuality and sexuality of the SCI person were shown to push the limits of tolerance of the observers. After desensitisation, there followed a discussion of personal sexual experiences from both the able-bodied and paraplegic participants. The education received by both groups was excellent. In a survey, all the participants reported they were glad they attended the workshop, 98% felt it was helpful to them, and 98% believed a similar programme should be offered to all SCI patients. A similar programme by Halsted et al. (1978) was also well received.

The goals of *individual* sexual counselling can be outlined by the PLISSIT model which has been used in SCI adults by King et al. (1985) and Madorsky and Dixon (1983). In this model, there are four levels of intervention: *P*ermission, *L*imited *I*nformation, *S*pecific *S*uggestions and *I*ntensive *T*herapy. Depending on the patients' level of understanding and comfort with the problems, they may receive brief counselling only, or they may need all levels proceeding through to lengthy intensive therapy.

In the permission phase (P), the topic of sexuality is first introduced. The counsellor discusses the baseline sexual function of the patient, any type of sexual activity that has been performed, and sexual interests or feelings of the patient. The patient is made comfortable that these feelings, interests and type of sexual activity are normal and can be practised.

Limited information is given regarding the anatomy, physiology, and reasonable expectations of performance derived from scientific experience. Along with the sexual issues, information regarding autonomic dysreflexia, urinary incontinence, and other matters as they relate to the sexual experience are discussed. Concepts regarding procreation and contraception can be introduced at this level.

In the next stage, suggestions to the male patient for his particular situation are given. For instance, if he is managed with an external urinary collection device, but does not empty his bladder fully, he might catheterise prior to intercourse to empty the bladder. For patients who have difficulty achieving erection, the use of vibrators, or the "stuff" technique (stuffing the flaccid penis into the vagina) may be helpful. Certain positions or type of activity such as oral-genital stimulation or the use of artificial devices to simulate erection may be suggested. Positions which cause autonomic hyperreflexia or incontinence are discovered and avoided.

For some patients and couples, the first three levels may not give adequate results, and intensive therapy may be necessary. This situation may be the result of monumental physical disability (e.g. ventilator-dependent quadriplegia), problems in communication and/or deep-seated aversion or anxieties which may or may not have been present prior to injury. This level of therapy is very individually designed and is best given by a psychologist, psychiatrist, social worker or other well-trained individual.

Treatment of Erectile Dysfunction

Penile Prosthesis Implantation

Although penile prosthesis implantation has been suggested to facilitate placement of an external urinary drainage appliance (VanArsdalen et al. 1981) the major indication in SCI patients is the treatment of erectile dysfunction. There has been experience with the use of semirigid (Rossier and Fam 1981), inflatable (Light and Scott 1981) and the newer self-contained inflatable devices (Green and Sloan 1986).

Although the semirigid prostheses have been used successfully, one series had an erosion rate of 25% (VanArsdalen et al. 1981). There may be a theoretical advantage in using the inflatable type to decrease the chance of erosion. With a semirigid device, an unnatural bend in the penis from sitting may cause pressure on the distal end of the rods in a SCI patient, in contrast to a patient with normal sensation who would simply readjust the penis on feeling the discomfort. Also, the newer non-distensible inflatable cylinders should be advantageous to prevent overinflation due to this lack of penile pain sensation.

Whatever type of prosthesis is selected, it would seem prudent to optimise urological and general health prior to implantation. We achieve stable bladder management without the use of indwelling catheters. The urine should be sterile and the patient free of decubiti prior to surgery to lessen the risk of infection. Strict aseptic technique should be used, as in any implantation of a prosthetic device. We generally use intravenous broad-spectrum antibiotics in the perioperative period.

Intracorporeal Injection Therapy

Since the first series showing that intracorporeal papaverine can cause penile erection (Virag 1982), there has been great interest in this area. There have been successes with injection of papaverine (Virag et al. 1984), phenoxybenzamine (Brindley 1983), and a combination of papaverine and phentolamine (Sidi et al. 1986). Bodner et al. (1987) successfully treated 19 of 20 SCI patients with papaverine alone or papaverine/phentolamine combination. The single failure was found to have abnormal penile venous drainage. Three patients had episodes of priapism resulting from doses of papaverine of 7.5–30 mg. All three patients subsequently responded to lower doses. Sidi et al. (1987) treated 66 SCI men with the same drug combinations. Fifty-two patients achieved functional erections and there were four cases of priapism. One patient in each of the above series developed induration near the injection sites. Autonomic dysreflexia was not seen.

Neurogenic patients respond well to intracavernosal injection therapy. The dosage needed tends to be lower than that needed for other impotent patients. To avoid priapism, we begin therapy with 15–20 mg of papaverine alone and increase progressively until the required dosage is reached. In an occasional patient, the addition of phentolamine is necessary. The injection is made in the lateral corporeal body with a 30-gauge needle. A constrictive band is placed at the base of the penis for two minutes and the injection site is held to avoid haematoma formation.

It should be kept in mind that the long-term effects of intracorporeal injections are not known. The ill-effects of priapism remain even in a carefully controlled programme. Because of these risks, and lack of Food and Drug Administration approval, the US manufacturer has recently modified the package insert to state that papaverine is not indicated for intracorporeal injection. Patients must be carefully selected, informed of the technique and possible risks, and followed closely.

Treatment of Ejaculatory Dysfunction

Intrathecal Neostigmine and Subcutaneous Physostigmine

Intrathecal neostigmine was first successfully used to cause ejaculation in an SCI man in 1947 by Guttman and he subsequently reported his experience with the procedure in 134 paraplegics and quadriplegics (Guttman and Walsh 1971). An average of 0.3 mg of neostigmine was found to cause decreased skeletal muscle spasticity, followed by sustained erection and repeated ejaculations over the next several hours. The procedure was successful in 58% of cases and more successful in spastic and complete lesions. Lesions below T10 had a lower success rate. In patients with lesions above T5, severe sustained autonomic dysreflexia occurred and there was a death of a C6-7 quadriplegic from the procedure. The danger of autonomic dysreflexia during the procedure has been noted by others (Rossier et al. 1971).

The first pregnancy by artificial insemination following intrathecal neostigmine was reported by Spira (1956). Since that time there have been only a few successes and it seems the risk–benefit ratio for this procedure may be too great, and we do not use it.

Chapelle et al. (1983) reported on the subcutaneous injection of physostigmine in 20 SCI men. Eight patients ejaculated on either the first or second trial. An anticholinergic medication, N-butylhyoscine bromide, was given to block the peripheral cholinergic effects. Autonomic dysreflexia was not seen, but orthostatic hypotension, tachycardia, nausea and vomiting were noted. Artificial insemination was not attempted in this group.

Vibratory Stimulation

Sobrero et al. (1965) reported using an electromechanical vibrator to cause ejaculation with a high success rate in groups of schizophrenics, normal men, infertility patients and anejaculatory men. There were two successful attempts of artificial insemination in one couple with one spontaneous abortion and one live birth. The first successful pregnancy by this technique in an SCI patient was performed by the patient at home and reported by Comarr (1970).

Brindley (1984) reported his experience with vibratory stimulation in 93 SCI patients. The success rate was 59%. There was only one success in 12 patients attempted in the first six months after injury and no successes in 19 patients who lacked reflex hip flexion. If those groups are disregarded, the success rate was 48/62 (77%). These data verify that this technique depends on an intact reflex from the genital afferents through the hypogastric sympathetic efferents. Autonomic dysreflexia was seen in high lesions and it continued in one patient for 10 minutes after the stimulation was removed. Seven pregnancies were achieved, mainly by intravaginal insemination.

Francois et al. (1980) used vibromassage on 50 patients with a 72% success rate. Any cutaneous lesions below T10, such as haemorrhoids or decubiti, were detrimental, possibly by altering the afferent signals reaching the spinal cord and modifying the ejaculatory reflex arc. Also noted was the ill-effect of urinary infection. The procedure was successful in 92% of patients with sterile urine and in 47% of patients with infection. Seven pregnancies were achieved in 16 couples, with four of these pregnancies achieved by intercourse following initial vibromassage.

The quality of semen in the series of Brindley and Francois tended to improve with successive ejaculations, especially in the motility. This was not the case in a recent series by Sarkarati et al. (1987).

Brindley (1984) employs a Ling 201 vibrator set at 80 Hz with an amplitude of 2.5 mm. The knob is placed on the ventral glans/frenulum area and applied until ejaculation occurs. Cycles of 3.5 minutes stimulation to 1.5 minutes rest are carried out for four cycles. The patients are stimulated in the supine position and pulled upright if dysreflexia occurs (for lesions above T5). Francois et al. (1980) begin at the base of the penis until erection occurs and then advance toward the glans. Some stimulations are carried out to achieve erection prior to vaginal intercourse and intravaginal ejaculation.

Electroejaculation

Horne et al. (1948) produced the first reported human electroejaculate with an insulated urethral sound as the electrode. They obtained an ejaculate with motile sperm in 9 of 18 patients with spinal cord injury.

Bensman and Kottke (1966) successfully used a rectal electrode to cause retrograde ejaculation in three of five patients. Autonomic dysreflexia was noted in one C6–7 quadriplegic. Frankel et al. (1974) reported a case of autonomic dysreflexia from electroejaculation and noted a simultaneous increase of plasma norepinephrine activity.

The first pregnancy from electroejaculated sperm was in 1975 (Thomas et al. 1975). Unfortunately, the baby died in the first day of life from transposition of the great vessels. Another pregnancy was reported by David et al. (1977), and the birth of a healthy girl by Francois et al. was noted in 1978. Martin et al. (1983) and Perkash et al. (1985) successfully obtained sperm by transrectal stimulation but felt the motility was too low to be appropriate for artificial insemination.

Brindley (1984) published his results of electroejaculation in 154 SCI patients. He obtained sperm in antegrade fashion in 69 and retrograde in 28 for total success rate of 62%. In contrast to vibratory stimulation, electroejaculation is successful in the spinal shock phase. He did feel, however, that electroejaculation or vibrator ejaculation would be unsuccessful in patients lacking the T11–L2 spinal segments, assuming that the presence of sympathetic cord outflow at this level was necessary for the success of the procedure. He also noted that retrograde ejaculate seemed to have poorer motility than antegrade. The quality of semen improved with successive electroejaculation trials. He had three pregnancies in his series from electroejaculated sperm. His technique used a finger electrode and he attempted to stimulate the obturator nerve area to achieve ejaculation (Brindley 1981).

We have had experience with electroejaculation in over 60 spinal cord injured males (unpublished data). The success rate at our centre for obtaining motile sperm is 70%. The first two pregnancies in the US were reported in 1987 (Bennett et al. 1987a) and we have had a total of seven pregnancies from 20 SCI men using the technique. Our technique involves stimulation via a hand-held rectal electrode. Following anoscopy, the electrode is inserted into the rectum with the electrodes facing anteriorly. The stimulation is given in a progressively increasing sine-wave pattern with frequency of approximately 5 seconds. The voltage is increased until ejaculation or a maximum of 30–35 volts (AC) is reached. Both antegrade and retrograde ejaculate is retrieved.

The specimens are centrifuged in insemination media to concentrate sperm and remove the urine. Next, either soft centrifugation with a density gradient or a "swim-up" technique is used to isolate motile sperm. These are reconcentrated in 0.2 ml of media and inseminated by intrauterine route at the appropriate time in the spouse's cycle. The timing is judged by basal body temperature charts and verified the day of insemination by ovarian ultrasound.

We have also noted an improvement in semen quality with successive electro-ejaculations. We have not, however, noted any worse prognosis for patients lacking sympathetic outflow. Our success in patients who are anejaculatory from retroperitoneal lymph node dissection (Bennett et al. 1987b) proves that an intact ejaculatory reflex arc via thoracolumbar sympathetics is not necessary for successful electroejaculation.

Conclusion

Medical care for the spinal cord injured has improved greatly in the last few decades. Improvements in rehabilitation encourage paraplegics and quadriplegics to find employment, participate in social events, and attempt to live fairly normal lives. Desire for sexual satisfaction of the patient and spouse and/or procreation are needs of many, if not the majority of SCI patients. With the use of standard and innovative techniques, many of these needs can now be satisfied.

In the medical management of the SCI man, we must take into consideration preserving future fertility. Aggressively pursuing a low-pressure bladder to keep patients free of infection, especially epididymitis, is a prime goal. To keep the possibility of use of vibratory stimulation available, rhizotomies for spasticity or pain must be avoided. To avoid inevitable retrograde ejaculation or obstruction of the ejaculatory ducts, transurethral resection of the bladder neck should be avoided. If these concerns are kept in mind, we may very well see fertility rates from the above mentioned procedures increase significantly.

References

Anderson TP, Cole TM (1975) Sexual counselling of the physically disabled. Postgrad Med 58: 117–123

Bennett CJ, Ayers JWT, Randolph JF et al. (1987a) Electroejaculation of paraplegic males followed by pregnancies. Fertil Steril 48: 1070–1072

Bennett CJ, Seager SWJ, McGuire EJ (1987b) Electroejaculation for recovery of semen after retroperitoneal lymph node dissection: case report. J Urol 137: 513–515

Bensman A, Kottke FJ (1966) Induced emission of sperm utilizing electrical stimulation of the seminal vesicles and vas deferens. Arch Phys Med Rehabil 47: 436–443

Benson GS, McConnell JA, Schmidt WA (1981) Penile polsters: functional structures or atherosclerotic changes? J Urol 125: 800–803

Bodner DR, Lindan R, Leffler E, Kursh ED, Resnick MI (1987) The application of intracavernous injection of vasoactive medications for erection in men with spinal cord injury. J Urol 138: 310–311

Bors E, Comarr AE (1960) Neurologic disturbance of sexual function with special reference to 529 patients with spinal cord injury. Urol Surv 10: 191–222

Bors E, Engle ET, Rosenquist RC, Holliger VH (1950) Fertility in paraplegic males – a preliminary report of endocrine studies. J Clin Endocrinol 10: 381–398

Brindley GS (1981) Electroejaculation: its technique, neurological implications and uses. J Neurol Neurosurg Psychiatry 44: 9–18

Brindley GS (1982) Deep scrotal temperature and the effect on it of clothing, air temperature, activity, posture and paraplegia. Br J Urol 54: 49–55

Brindley GS (1983) Cavernosal alpha-blockage: a new technique for investigating and treating erectile impotence. Br J Psychiatry 143: 332–334

Brindley GS (1984) The fertility of men with spinal injuries. Paraplegia 22: 337–348

Catanzarite VA, Ferguson JE, Weinstein CS (1984) Clinical management of spinal cord injury. Obstet Gynecol 64: 598–599 letter

Chapelle PA, Blanquart F, Puech AJ, Held JP (1983) Treatment of anejaculation in the total paraplegic by subcutaneous injection of physostigmine. Paraplegia 21: 30–36

Cole TM (1975a) Sexuality and physical disabilities. Arch Sex Behav 4: 389–403

Cole TM (1975b) Reaction of the rehabilitation team to patients with sexual problems. Arch Phys Med Rehabil 56: 10–11

Cole TM, Stevens MR (1975) Rehabilitation professionals and Sexual Counseling for Spinal Cord Injured Adults. Arch Sex Behav 4: 631–638

Cole TM, Chilgren R, Rosenberg P (1973) A new programme of sex education and counselling for spinal cord injured adults and health care professionals. Paraplegia 11: 111–124

Comarr AE (1966) Observations on menstruation and pregnancy among female spinal cord injury patients. Paraplegia 3: 263–271

Comarr AE (1970) Sexual function among patients with spinal cord injury. Urol Int 25: 134–168

Comarr AE (1971) Sexual concepts in traumatic cord and cauda equina lesions. J Urol 106: 375–378

Conine TA, Disher CS, Gilmore SL, Fischer BAP (1979) Physical therapists' knowledge of sexuality of adults with spinal cord injury. Phys Ther 59: 395–398

Conti G (1952) Erection of the human penis and its morphological-vascular bases (in French). Acta Anat (Basel) 14: 217–262

David A, Ohry A, Rozin R (1977) Spinal cord injuries: male fertility aspects. Paraplegia 15: 11–14

Deyoe FS (1972) Marriage and family patterns with long-term spinal cord injury. Paraplegia 10: 219–224

Domer FR, Wessler G, Brown RL, Charles HC (1978) Involvement of the sympathetic nervous system in the urinary bladder internal sphincter and in penile erection in the anesthetized cat. Invest Urol 15: 404–407

Dorr LD, Brody MJ (1967) Hemodynamic mechanism of erection in the canine penis. Am J Physiol 213: 1526–1531

Eckhardt C (1863) Quoted in Siroky and Krane (1983)

Francois N, Maury M, Jouannet D, David G, Vacant J (1978) Electroejaculation of a complete paraplegic followed by pregnancy. Paraplegia 16: 248–251

Francois N, Lichtenberger JM, Jouannet P, Desert JF, Maury M (1980) L'éjaculation par le vibromassage chez le paraplegique à propos de 50 cas avec 7 grossesses. Ann Med Phys 23: 24–36

Frankel HL, Mathias CJ, Walsh JJ (1974) Blood pressure, plasma catecholamines and prostaglandins during artificial erection in a male tetraplegic. Paraplegia 12: 205–211

Goller H, Paeslack V (1972) Pregnancy damage and birth-complications in the children of paraplegic women. Paraplegia 10: 213–217

Green BG, Sloan SL (1986) Penile prosthesis in spinal cord injured patients: combined psychosexual counselling and surgical regimen. Paraplegia 24: 167–172

Greenspoon JS, Paul RH (1986) Paraplegia and quadriplegia: special considerations during pregnancy and labor and delivery. Am J Obstet Gynecol 155: 738–741

Grynbaum BB, Kaplan LI, Lloyd KE (1963) Quoted in Teal JC, Athelstan GT (1975) Sexuality and spinal cord injury: some psychosocial considerations. Arch Phys Med Rehabil 56: 264–268

Guttman L (1964) The married life of paraplegics and tetraplegics. Paraplegia 2: 182–188

Guttman L, Walsh JJ (1971) Prostigmine assessment of fertility in spinal man. Paraplegia 9: 39–51

Guttman L, Frankel HL, Paeslack V (1965) Cardiac irregularities during labour in paraplegic women. Paraplegia 3: 144–151

Halsted LS, Halsted MG, Salhoot JT, Stock DD, Sparks RW (1978) Sexual attitudes, behavior and satisfaction for able-bodied and disabled participants attending workshops in human sexuality. Arch Phys Med Rehabil 59: 497–501

Hayes PJ, Krishnan KR, Diver MJ, Hipkin LF, Davis JC (1979) Testicular endocrine function in paraplegic men. Clin Endocrinol 11: 549–552

Horne HW, Paull DP, Munro D (1948) Fertility studies in the human male with traumatic injuries of the spinal cord and cauda equina. N Engl J Med 239: 959–961

Jackson RW (1972) Sexual rehabilitation after cord injury. Paraplegia 10: 10–55

Karacan I, Aslan C, Hirshkowitz M (1983) Erectile mechanisms in man. Science 220: 1080–1082

Kedia KR (1983) Ejaculation and emission: normal physiology, dysfunction and therapy. In: Krane RJ, Siroky MB, Goldstein I (eds) Male sexual dysfunction. Little Brown, Boston, pp 37–51

Kedia KR, Markland C, Fraley EE (1975) Sexual function following high retroperitoneal lymphadenectomy. J Urol 114: 237–239

Kikuchi TA, Skowsky WR, El-Toraei I, Swerdloff R (1976) The pituitary-gonadal axis in spinal cord injury. Fertil Steril 27: 1142–1145

King NJ, Klein RM, Remenyi AG (1985) Sexual counselling with spinal cord injured persons. Aust Fam Physician 14: 47–51

Krane RJ, Siroky MB (1981) Neurophysiology of erection. Urol Clin North Am 8: 91–102

Leriche A, Berard E, Vauzelle JL et al. (1977) Histological and hormonal testicular changes in spinal cord patients. Paraplegia 15: 274–279

Light JK, Scott FB (1981) Management of neurogenic impotence with inflatable penile prosthesis. Urology 17: 341–343

Madorsky JGB, Dixon TP (1983) Rehabilitation aspects of human sexuality. West J Med 139: 174–176

Martin, DE, Warner H, Crenshaw TL, Crenshaw RT, Shapiro CE, Perkash I (1983) Initiation of erection and semen release by rectal probe electrostimulation (RPE). J Urol 129: 637–642

Morales PA, Hardin J (1958) Scrotal and testicular temperature studies in paraplegics. J Urol 79: 972–975

Morley JE, Distiller LA, Lissoos I et al. (1979) Testicular function in patients with spinal cord damage. Horm Metab Res 11: 679–682

Munro D, Horne HW, Paull DP (1948) The effect of injury to the spinal cord and cauda equina on the sexual potency of men. N Engl J Med 239: 903–911

Newman HF, Northrup JD (1981) Mechanisms of human penile erection: an overview. Urology 17: 399–408

Nilsson S, Obrant KO, Persson PS (1968) Changes in the testis parenchyma caused by acute nonspecific epididymitis. Fertil Steril 19: 748–757

Ohry A, Peleg D, Goldman J, David A, Rozin R (1978) Sexual function, pregnancy and delivery in spinal cord injured women. Gynecol Obstet Invest 9: 281–291

Ottesen B, Wagner G, Virag R, Fahrenkrug J (1984) Penile erection: possible role for vasoactive intestinal polypeptide as a neurotransmitter. Br Med J 288: 9–11

Perkash I, Martin DE, Warner H, Blank MS, Collins DC (1985) Reproductive biology of paraplegics: results of semen collection, testicular biopsy and serum hormone evaluation. J Urol 134: 284–288

Phelps G, Brown M, Chen J et al. (1983) Sexual experience and plasma testosterone levels in male veterans after spinal cord injury. Arch Phys Med Rehabil 64: 47–52

Robertson DNS (1972) Pregnancy and labour in the paraplegic. Paraplegia 10: 209–212

Root WS, Bard P (1947) The mechanism of feline erection through sympathetic pathways with some remark on sexual behavior after deafferentation of the genitalia. Am J Physiol 150: 80–90

Rossier AB, Fam BA (1984) Indication and results of semirigid penile prostheses in spinal cord injury patients: long term followup. J Urol 131: 59–62

Rossier AB, Ziegler WH, Duchosal PW, Meylan J (1971) Sexual function and dysreflexia. Paraplegia 9: 51–59

Sarkarati M, Rossier AB, Fam BA (1987) Experience in vibratory and electroejaculation techniques in spinal cord injury patients: a preliminary report. J Urol 138: 59–62

Sidi AA, Cameron JS, Duffy LM, Lange PH (1986) Intracavernous drug-induced erections in the management of male erectile dysfunction: experience with 100 patients. J Urol 135: 704–706

Sidi AA, Cameron JS, Dyksta DD, Reinberg Y, Lange PH (1987) Vasoactive intracavernous pharmacotherapy for the treatment of erectile impotence in men with spinal cord injury. J Urol 138: 539–542

Siroky MB, Krane RJ (1983) Neurophysiology of erection. In: Krane RJ, Siroky MB, Goldstein I (eds) Male sexual dysfunction. Little Brown, Boston, pp 9–20

Sobrero AJ, Stearns HE, Blari JH (1965) Technic for the induction of ejaculation in humans. Fertil Steril 16: 765–767

Spielman FJ (1984) Parturient with spinal cord transection: complications of autonomic hyperreflexia. Obstet Gynecol 64: 147

Spira R (1956) Artificial insemination after intrathecal injection of neostigmine in a paraplegic. Lancet 1: 670–671

Talbot HS (1955) The sexual function in paraplegia. J Urol 73: 91–100

Talbot HS (1971) Psychosocial aspects of sexuality in spinal cord injury patients. Paraplegia 9: 37–39

Thomas AJ (1983) Ejaculatory dysfunction. Fertil Steril 39: 445–454

Thomas RJS, McLeish G, McDonald IA (1975) Electroejaculation of the paraplegic male followed by pregnancy. Med J Aust 2: 798–799

Tsuji I, Nakajima F, Morimoto J, Nounada Y (1961) The sexual function in patients with spinal cord injury. Urol Int 12: 270–280

Wagenknect LF (1985) Causes of obstruction of the male reproductive tract. In: Wagenknect LF (ed) Microsurgery in urology. Thieme, New York

Weinberg JS (1982) Human sexuality and spinal cord injury. Neurosurg Clin North Am 17: 407–419

VanArsdalen KN, Klein FA, Hackler RH, Brady SM (1981) Penile implants in spinal cord injury patients for maintaining external appliances. J Urol 126: 331–332

Virag R (1982) Intracavernous injection of papavarine for erectile failure. Lancet 2: 938 (letter)

Virag R, Frydman D, Legman M, Virag H (1984) Intracavernous injection of papaverine as a diagnostic and therapeutic method in erectile failure. Angiology 35: 79–87

Young BK, Katz M, Klein SA (1983) Pregnancy after spinal cord injury: altered maternal and fetal response to labor. Obstet Gynecol 62: 59–63

Zeitlin AB, Cottrell TL, Lloyd FA (1957) Sexology of the paraplegic male. Fertil Steril 8: 337–344

Psychological Considerations

C.A. Glass

Introduction

Sexuality has been a central concern of psychologists, at least as far back as Freud (1856–1939), whose concept of sexual energy (Eros) formed a cornerstone of his general theory of human behaviour. Difficulties relating to performance of sexual activity have similarly been noted throughout the development of understanding of sexual behaviour, as can be seen in the material of workers such as Havelock Ellis (1858–1939), and von Kraft-Ebbing (1840–1902).

Therapeutic intervention regarding such difficulties, however, tended to meet with little success until the development of the work of Masters and Johnson (1966). These authors produced a major breakthrough in sex research with their use of direct observation and physiological recording of sexual activity. More recently researchers such as Karacan (1969) and Fisher et al. (1976) have expanded upon these earlier investigations to examine methods of objective assessment of sexual functioning as aids in the differential diagnosis of sexual difficulties.

The assessment and treatment of sexual functioning and dysfunction in those with spinal injuries has benefited from both the development of these techniques and the investigations of physiological function by pioneers such as Bors and Comarr (1960) and Brindley et al. (1974).

The aim of this section of Chapter 7 is to summarise the current status of assessment of sexual dysfunction in both females and males who have experienced spinal trauma, and then to explore methods of treatment which have been shown to have some success in overcoming those difficulties which have a psychogenic basis.

Assessment of Female Sexual Behaviour and Dysfunction

One of the least researched areas of spinal injury has been the effect on female sexuality. There is, however, a substantial amount of literature concerning female sexuality in general, and this may serve as an indicator of the abilities and needs of those with spinal injury. Much of this literature relates to the frequency and type of sexual behaviour in which women engage (Kinsey et al. 1953; Fisher 1973), whilst a similar volume examines the frequency and type of sexual dysfunctions which women experience (Kilmann 1978).

However, the cultural and social taboos surrounding the expression of sexuality by women make sample bias an obvious concern in the information currently available. It remains unclear what factors are associated with arousal in women, other than the overgeneralisation that it is likely to be an interaction between physiological factors influencing arousal, and situational and/or interpersonal factors.

There have been reports published recently (Geer et al. 1974; Beck et al. 1983) which have begun to examine arousal in women using a vaginal plethysmograph. This device is similar in shape to a tampon and detects changes in opacity in the vagina caused by increases in blood flow during arousal. Whilst the physiological mechanisms underlying vaginal vasocongestion are not understood, the phenomenon has been used as a measure of arousal in women, and there is some evidence to suggest that vaginal blood flow does increase during exposure to erotic stimuli and masturbation (Fisher et al. 1983).

Whilst the current understanding of sexual arousal in women is low, what remains clear is that sexual expression and need are as great in women with spinal trauma as they are in men with similar conditions. Money (1960) interviewed 7 women, aged between 21 and 65, whose time since trauma ranged from 6 months to almost 14 years. Although 3 had been non-orgasmic prior to trauma and although 2 of 3 who had attempted intercourse reported negative feelings, 2 further women reported pleasurable sexual feelings as a result of breast stimulation.

The most comprehensive study currently available was conducted by Bregman (1975). In common with most research in this area it contains serious methodological problems. All of the sample of 31 women reported that they had engaged in sexual activity post-trauma; 27 reported that they still experienced vaginal lubrication, and most subjects considered that spinal trauma had not affected sexual arousal or lubrication, although all experienced diminution of vaginal sensation.

Less research has perhaps been published concerning this group than for men with spinal injuries because of the smaller number of cases of trauma which involve women. Trieschmann (1980) reports that in the band of 15 to 29 year olds, which constitute 60% of spinal injuries in the USA, 82% are male and 18% female. It has also been suggested (Bardlach and Anderson 1979) that women have lower adjustment difficulties because the mechanics of female sexual activity do not traditionally require as much activity as that of males. However, whilst this may be true (given the current state of knowledge concerning normal sexual activity) it is a statement based on expectation rather than objective observation. It is unclear, for example, whether couples where the female adopted superior positions during sexual activity prior to trauma have experienced any alteration in either the quality or quantity of sexual activity due to the subsequent need for the male partner to adopt this position.

However, it is important not to view sexual behaviour in isolation as intercourse for most couples tends to arise as an expression of the overall quality of their relationship. Investigators have attempted to evaluate individual factors associated with overall quality of interpersonal relationships, such as self concept (Nagler 1950), and body image (Ryan 1961). Fink et al. (1969), for example, studied the impact of severe mobility impairment on sexual interaction in a group of disabled married women, including those who had experienced spinal trauma. Sexual satisfaction correlated significantly with overall marital satisfaction, and for their partners there was a similar correlation but this failed to reach significance. Although this latter study reinforces the need to take the views of both partners into account in assessing experience of sexual functioning, the general lack of control groups and reliance on self report in studies of this kind make estimation of the reliability of the data somewhat difficult.

In terms of treatment of sexual dysfunctions which are raised by women, the most frequent difficulties which arise concern a perceived overall lack of pleasure by both partners and, less commonly, an inability to allow penetration due to spasticity.

Couples often report that they do not feel anything during sexual intercourse, or that the whole process fails to provide any real pleasure. The commonest causes of these forms of difficulty are inappropriate expectation and/or inadequate exploration of individual need. Such difficulties frequently arise due to problems in communication, and this issue will be dealt with in the section on treatment of male psychosexual dysfuction, as it is common to both.

The experience of spasticity is common in spinal trauma. It is the involuntary movement (jerking) of muscles which occur because of reflex activity in the spine below the level of the lesion and which, because they are no longer regulated by the brain, become exaggerated. A number of women have reported that their spasticity results in their partners being unable to penetrate either because the overall level of activity is too great, or because the spasticity results in their legs being brought together making penetration impossible. Discussion about the sexual activity prior to penetration often leads to an alleviation of the difficulty; if the condition continues to interfere with sexual activity, medication or surgery may be recommended by the spinal consultant.

It is important to remember that although sensation in the vagina is reduced or absent, those women who ovulate can still conceive and give natural birth to their children (Gutmann 1964; Comarr 1966). For this reason, advice on contraception should be given at an early stage during rehabilitation. Single women may not wish to start a family and married women often want to allow some time following discharge to adjust to being at home.

However, it may be difficult for the woman to find a method of contraception which is suitable to her. Birth control pills are usually not recommended because of the associated risk of blood clotting, and a diaphragm may be practically difficult to use, particularly by those with higher level lesions. Whilst intrauterine devices present few problems for women with spinal injuries, they are not always well favoured. The use of a condom by the partner is therefore a commonly used alternative. If the woman has no desire to conceive, sterilisation of either partner may be considered, but this should only be entered into following comprehensive physical and psychological investigation.

In summary, the present understanding of female sexual dysfuction following spinal trauma is marred by the paucity of adequately controlled, methodologically rigorous investigations. Techniques of vaginal plethysmography may produce important information in the future, though the experience of sexual pleasure is considered to arise out of a combination of physiological, interpersonal and situational determinants. In order to facilitate women to raise concerns over sexuality following trauma it is important that the initial rehabilitation environment is supportive of the expression of such views. It is the author's experience that, particularly for younger women, their ability to have children in the future is one of the commonest worries raised in the first few weeks following trauma. Furthermore, at this time, objective and compassionate explanation of the factors associated with sexuality usually provides a foundation for couples to come forward for assistance if difficulties are experienced once the injured person returns home.

Assessment of Male Psychosexual Disorders

Given the increased frequency with which younger men experience spinal trauma, the mechanics associated with sexual arousal, and the cultural acceptance of the expression of sexuality by men, it is understandable that they seek assistance with sexual difficulties more readily than women. However, care must be taken by all therapists in accepting such a generalisation as applicable in all cases; it must be remembered that individual variation will make some men more likely to express concerns than others. There is evidence to suggest that the experience of any form of severe trauma affects self confidence (Beard and Sampson 1981), the individual's perception of masculinity (Shambaugh et al. 1967), and can result in role reversal in some cases (Glass et al. 1988), such that the partner takes on the traditional male role of provider. In such situations it is to be expected that sexual functioning may become reduced, even in situations where the individual has functional vascular, neurological and hormonal systems. A recent review article (Abrams 1981) examined the available spinal trauma literature concerning marital stability, sexual interaction, and marital satisfaction, and concluded that:

1. The incidence of marital termination following trauma does not appear to increase in general, but low income and unemployment appear to be predictive of separation or divorce in a sub-group of paraplegics.
2. There is a paucity of literature concerned with estimation of pre- and post-morbid sexual activity and, without this, estimates of current sexual activity become meaningless.
3. So few studies have examined changes in marital satisfaction following trauma that it cannot be concluded that trauma has a detrimental effect.

The quality of current psychosocial and demographic research means that definition of the causal relationships between trauma, environment and the development of marital and sexual dysfunction cannot be made. There does, however, appear to be agreement amongst professionals involved in spinal trauma that interpersonal, psychosocial and psychosexual needs, together with physical and medical conditions, are important concerns in rehabilitation (Sha'ked and Flynn 1978; Conine 1984).

When an individual patient presents with erectile difficulties, the initial problem for the therapist is to decide upon the cause of the difficulty. The ability to obtain an erection is essentially a vascular response, although there remains some controversy surrounding the actual mechanism of erection (Wagner 1981; Benson et al. 1983).

Not only is an adequate blood supply necessary to initiate and maintain an erection, but intact neurological pathways must also be maintained. However, it is recognised that alpha-adrenergic blockade will produce erection; it would therefore appear justified to assume that the penis is continuously stimulated via the alpha-adrenergic sympathetic pathways and that disruption of these pathways, or stimulation of the pelvic splanchnic or hypogastric fibres, which are antagonistic to them, will produce sustained erection (Polack et al. 1981).

Various studies have examined the effects of denervation at different levels of the spinal cord (Weiss 1972), and indicate that erection can be mediated through either sacral (parasympathetic) or thoracolumbar (sympathetic) segments of the spinal cord; erections resulting from penile stimulation are mediated by a sacral reflex arc, whilst erections which arise due to psychogenic stimuli can be mediated through either the sympathetic or parasympathetic systems via impulses from the cortex. Bors and Comarr (1960) found that approximately 90% of patients with complete spinal cord lesions above the level of the sacral cord reported having erections following stimulation of the genitalia. However, this information was derived from questioning the patients and not from direct observation of erectile change.

Psychogenic erections, or those resulting from thoughts and feelings, are reported to occur less frequently following spinal trauma. Brindley (1981) noted that those with lesion levels below T9 should be able to experience some degree of psychogenic erection, whilst those with lesions at T8 cannot be discounted. Brindley (1984), combining data from two earlier studies, concluded that 63% of men with non-cervical lesions were able to obtain reflex but not psychogenic erections. Of those able to obtain psychogenic erections, 89% were able to achieve coitus. For complete cervical lesions, almost half reported being able to achieve coitus, of which 49% were by reflex erections.

The ability to experience ejaculation is something which is also severely affected by spinal trauma, though it has been shown recently to be preserved in a greater number of paraplegics and tetraplegics than was previously supposed (Francois et al. 1980). For complete lesions, ejaculation without the aid of a vibrator has been reported in 4 of 110 cervical lesions, 3 of 78 upper thoracic lesions, and 41 of 416 lower thoracic and lumbar lesions. The use of vibrators greatly increases these numbers, with Brindley (1981) reporting 10 of 11 cervical, 27 of 41 T1 to T10, and 2 of 9 T11 to L1 cases able to do so. Due to the small amount of neurological sparing required to leave such processes functional, incomplete lesions have a much higher incidence of erectile and ejaculatory ability than those with complete lesions.

The available data would support the hypothesis that sexual functioning is linked to lesion level, and that incomplete lesions tend to have a better prognosis for adequate sexual functioning. However, the majority of studies which have examined sexual functioning have relied on self report or questionnaire responses. There are few studies available in the spinal cord injury literature which explore the use of objective methods of erectile assessment as a method of differential diagnosis for expressed secondary impotence, although the procedures are now well established.

Differential Diagnosis of Impotence

Most texts recommend a two-phased procedure for the differential diagnosis of psychogenic and organic impotence (e.g. LoPiccolo and Heiman 1975):

1. History and physical examination for evidence of conditions known to be associated with impotence.
2. Noting from the patient's history signs of psychogenic impotence, such as gradual deterioration in erectile ability, occurrence in specific situations only, and some residual response (such as the presence of erections upon waking).

However, there are a number of limitations to this procedure, particularly in dealing with males following trauma. For example, conditions such as spinal trauma are known to be associated with a high incidence of impotence, and it may be assumed that the person will therefore have such a difficulty without definitive support for such a hypothesis being obtained, if the physical examination procedure is not carried out comprehensively. Furthermore, the accuracy of diagnosis of organic impotence is questionable since direct information concerning the neurological and vascular causes of impotence are not proven. Therapists must instead rely upon information that has been largely derived from clinical study and individual observation. The accuracy of diagnosis for psychogenic impotence is questionable because in practice any patient who does not exhibit obvious physical abnormalities usually receives such a diagnosis. Finally, the timing of the assessment of erectile functioning is important as it is known that there is suppression of reflex activity below the level of injury for a number of weeks (Amelar and Dubin 1982). These authors suggest that any deficits which are shown to be present after six months post-injury are likely to be permanent, and so it must be inferred that assessment of erectile functioning is best undertaken after this period of time.

When the methods of treating impotence were limited in effectiveness, accurate diagnosis of the cause of the problem was relatively unimportant. However, with the current availability of physiological and psychological procedures to assess and treat impotence, the need for a more comprehensive and reliable diagnostic procedure is now imperative.

Development of Nocturnal Penile Tumescence (NPT) Assessment

Zuckerman (1971), in a review of the available literature, showed that genital measurement provides the only objective assessment of sexual arousal in the male. A number of devices have been developed to assess both change in circumference (e.g. Barlow et al. 1970) and penile volume (e.g. Freund et al. 1965), with more recent investigators examining measures of penile rigidity (Virag et al. 1985).

The existence of erectile response during sleep was noted by Ohlmeyer et al. (1944). Fisher et al. (1965) conducted the first study to make simultaneous all-night recordings of eye movements during dreaming activity (REM sleep) and erectile change. Full or partial erections were found to occur in 95% of the 86 periods of REM sleep observed in 17 subjects.

Karacan (1970) was the first to suggest that the study of NPT might provide a useful clinical tool for the differential diagnosis of impotence. In summarising the results of screening over 300 cases (impotent diabetics, psychogenically impotent men, and age-matched normal controls), NPT was found to be normal in the psychogenic cases and absent in the organic cases.

Other authors have urged the need for caution in using NPT results to differentially diagnose organic and psychogenic impotence, for both theoretical and technical reasons.

Karacan (1970) noted that NPT was impaired or absent in normal men during REM periods which were associated with dreams considered to contain high anxiety content. However, the reliance on subsequent self report makes such interpretation open to question. What does seem clear is that there is a marked discrepancy between the quality of recording on the first night of assessment and those taken on subsequent nights. This "first night" effect is assumed to be due to the novelty of the situation and the procedure being undertaken, and most authors tend to remove these data from subsequent analysis.

Other authors have urged caution because of the differences in erectile response which can be attributed to the position in which recording devices are placed on the penis, with those placed at the base of the penis producing larger circumference changes in comparison with those placed immediately behind the glans (Fisher et al. 1979). There is, therefore, general agreement among investigators that the only accurate method of determining the sufficiency of erectile change for penetration is to observe it directly and test the rigidity. However, an adequate observation of this is probably the most difficult stage to examine as it is often not possible to time the awakening of the patient so that the observed erection is sufficiently rigid for penetration.

Marshall et al. (1981) adopted two rules which could be used to categorise correctly the vast majority of their impotent patients. They used physical examination and history of the presenting problem to assign 20 patients complaining of impotence into four groups: purely organic, purely psychological, mixed aetiology, and uncertain diagnosis. They then carried out NPT assessment over two nights.

They concluded that NPT could differentiate 80% of the patients into organic or psychogenic if they applied the rule that a change in erection circumference greater than 11.5 mm over baseline indicated psychogenic difficulties, whilst a change of less than or equal to 11.5 mm indicated organic difficulties. This procedure correctly identified 9 out of 10 organic cases but only 7 out of 10 psychogenic cases. Ninety-five per cent of cases could be correctly classified if they also applied the rule that two full NPTs or less implied organicity, whilst three or more implied psychogenic difficulties. Ten out of 10 organics were correctly identified and 9 out of 10 psychogenic cases.

However, Karacan et al. (1978) noted that psychogenic impotence was always caused by a complex interaction between psychological and physiological factors. NPT assessment must not, therefore, be considered as a procedure to determine whether any individual can equal values for frequency or duration of full or partial tumescence, but as a procedure to demonstrate that the patient has sufficient physiological capacity to obtain an erection of sufficient rigidity for penetration, and to maintain it for a period of time sufficient for satisfactory intercourse.

On the basis of this postulate, Wasserman et al. (1980) operationally defined impotence as psychogenic if:

The patient has one or more full erections during the nights of the NPT recording, confirmed by direct observation, to be adequate for vaginal penetration and maintained with this degree of rigidity for five or more consecutive minutes.

The operational use of this definition has been shown to have some reliability in further investigations (Glass et al. 1988; Glass 1989).

Only one study has so far been published which has begun to examine the presence of NPT following spinal trauma. Lamid (1985) examined NPT response in 24 patients – 12 paraplegic and 12 tetraplegic – each group containing 6 complete and 6 incomplete lesions. Recordings were made of the number of NPT episodes, the duration of each episode and the increase over baseline circumference measured in mm.

Those in each group with incomplete lesions were found to obtain greater increase in tumescence than those in their group with complete lesions, but the difference was not significant.

Mean duration of erectile episodes was found to be statistically significant with tetraplegics maintaining erections for 14.9 minutes, and paraplegics for 4.75 minutes. Similarly, the mean increase over baseline circumference of 13.3 mm for tetraplegics and 4.25 mm for paraplegics was also statistically significant.

However, whilst there are some methodological errors in the study which make interpretation of the results difficult (e.g. the level of trauma which resulted in the categorisation into the two groups is not clear) the author's conclusion that NPT is a valuable method to aid differential diagnosis of secondary impotence appears warranted.

Treatment of Psychosexual Dysfunction

Treatment in this area has historically been conducted outside the mainstream of academic psychology, with most therapists being clinicians with little interest in producing objective assessment of the variables associated with effectiveness. It was not until 1958, when Wolpe published *Psychotherapy by reciprocal inhibition*, that investigators began to examine the application of conditioning principles to the treatment of various sexual dysfunctions.

Such techniques only received wider attention following the publication of *Human sexual inadequacy* by Masters and Johnson (1970), wherein these procedures were expanded to form the basis of a comprehensive treatment approach.

The theoretical framework adopted by clinicians continues to be simply a matter of personal preference. Jehu (1979) in his book *Sexual dysfunction* begins on a personal note by stating that he considers himself to be a behaviour therapist, not a sex therapist, as he applies essentially the same approach whether he is dealing with a sexual or any other kind of psychological difficulty. It is this author's contention, in support of this view, that the application of behaviourism to the assessment and treatment of sexual dysfunction allows for more objective assessment of outcome.

A fundamental issue which does require thought before beginning to provide psychosexual support is the therapist's own perceptions and feelings about sexual activity. Potential therapists must have a comprehensive knowledge of the literature pertaining to normal and dysfunctional activity, must examine and resolve their own prejudices, and in the field of spinal injuries have a sound understanding of the physical and psychosocial implications on both the individual, the family and their role in society. Whilst such a statement should not need to be made, the present author is aware of numerous instances where such issues have not been resolved. Cases have been referred, after having been seen by numerous therapists, where, for example, differential diagnosis of the presenting condition has not been attempted, or couples have been refused therapy once it became clear that they were involved in homosexual relationships.

One of the first difficulties which frequently needs to be addressed in therapy is the nature of the presenting difficulty. Following spinal injury, patients are more likely to attribute any change in functioning to the trauma, such that it is often difficult for patients to accept that their difficulty may not have a physical basis. In helping the patient to overcome this it is often helpful to go through each of the assessment procedures undertaken in turn, where possible showing the person the original data and explaining what each means. Patients are often concerned that referral to a clinical psychologist means they have a mental difficulty, which often arises because the public rarely understands the distinction between a psychologist and psychiatrist.

Related to this issue is the need to involve the partner in therapy. Behaviourists view psychological problems as ways of responding in certain situations which are either problematic for individuals themselves, or for the people around them. The inability to experience arousal, or the inability to obtain an erection in the absence of any physical abnormality, are therefore seen as specific behavioural difficulties. As such behaviours are learnt they must therefore be amenable to change, provided the conditions which led to the difficulty are modified in some way. In sexual dysfunction it is considered that some aspect associated with the interaction whilst making love acts as an aversive stimulus to either or both partners. It may well be, for example, that a male spouse does not approach his injured wife for fear of inducing spasms. Similarly, the inability of a spinal injured male to obtain an erection may be due to feelings of inadequacy, or feelings of embarrassment associated with the possibility of urine leakage.

Whilst involving both partners in therapy is considered important, and is supported by research data from other areas of disability (e.g. Cooper 1969), there are a small number of cases where the sexual problem might not be seen as a relationship difficulty. The inability to function sexually due to strict moral or religious upbringing may result due to the individual never having learned the cues or techniques involved in foreplay or love making. In one such case the author provided initial therapy to the individual, which was only extended to include a partner some years later, once he had become established in a stable relationship.

However, in most cases, if patients and spouses are to begin to overcome their specific psychosexual difficulty it is important that communication is as accessible and unambiguous as possible. One of the primary aims of therapy is therefore to provide an atmosphere which is conducive to the exploration of the potential factors associated with the expressed difficulty in such a way which provokes the least amount of anxiety for either partner.

The purpose of early sessions is to establish a comprehensive description of the presenting difficulty, and to obtain some understanding of the antecedents, or those personal and interactional issues involved in bringing the expressed difficulty about. Once such information is gained it is then possible to begin to examine those issues which are responsible for the maintenance of the problem. A number of authors have produced checklists of the information normally required for the production of a clear analysis of a presenting difficulty. One of the most comprehensive is produced as an appendix to the book written by Jehu (1979). Whilst the use of such checklists can appear mechanical and inflexible, it must be stressed that not all areas will be relevant in all cases, and it is the role of the behaviour therapist to select those which are of most relevance to each individual case.

Having obtained a detailed account of the factors associated with the presented difficulty, there are a number of specific treatment strategies which can then be undertaken. As therapists use different theoretical approaches, treatments offered vary considerably, although only a behavioural perspective will be offered in this chapter.

However, regardless of therapeutic preference, what does appear to be important (though the theoretical data in support of this view are limited) is that graduated sexual experiences in treatment are preferable to, and therefore presumably more effective than, non-graduated experiences.

Bandura (1969) suggested a number of reasons why this should be the case. Non-graduated experiences may increase the patient's anxiety to the point whereby exposure becomes aversive, leading to future avoidance of exposure to sexual activity. Another important factor associated with gradual exposure is that it means both the therapist and the patient have a greater degree of control over what occurs in the therapeutic situation.

What remains unclear is the comparative effectiveness of the single therapist, or the use of co-therapists in such treatment approaches. Masters and Johnson (1970) noted that

> Definitive laboratory experience supports the concept that a more successful clinical approach to the problem of sexual dysfunctions can be made by the dual-sex team of therapists that by an individual male or female therapist.

Other clinicians argue that co-therapy is not necessary; Kaplan (1974) states that therapists can be trained to understand the sexuality of opposite-sexed patients, whilst McCarthy (1973) argued that co-therapy is more expensive in terms of both time and money.

The arguments for and against the use of co-therapists is essentially an empirical one and should not be conducted on a cost–benefit basis. The important issue is therefore whether co-therapy teams increase the effectiveness of psychosexual counselling, and the available literature would appear to suggest not.

Franks and Wilson (1974) stated that no research actually supports Masters and Johnson's claims and that clinical evidence suggested that single male therapists can successfully treat female dysfunctions, citing the works of Brady (1969) and Wolpin (1969) to support their case.

Clement and Schmidt (1983) in an examination of 202 couples used three different treatment formats:

1. *Two therapists, long term*. Male and female therapist, two sessions per week for 35–40 sessions.
2. *One therapist, long term*. Male or female therapist, two sessions per week for 35–40 sessions.

3. *Two therapists, intensive.* Male and female therapist, daily sessions for three weeks, 16 sessions.

They concluded that there were no significant differences between one versus two therapists, though there was a slight trend towards better results from long-term therapy as opposed to intensive therapy.

In a review of five sexual counselling programmes for people with spinal injuries, Schuler (1982) concluded that there were a number of factors which appeared common. The initial stage of most programmes was the presentation of information regarding sexual function and the resultant changes following trauma. The examination of prejudice and the exploration of myths surrounding sexuality were approached at the same time as the information was being presented. A major goal of all programmes was for the injured person to redefine their sexuality, exploring the compensations which had to be made for the loss of function in various parts of the body, and redefining those areas which produced the greatest degree of arousal. As each group progressed there was increasing emphasis placed on practical activity and exploration of the individual's needs.

The provision of such support groups in the UK undoubtedly falls short of the number available in the USA. However, it remains unclear whether exploration of sexuality in a large group format is the most efficient way of disseminating information, or whether individual couple therapy enables both the therapist and those engaged in therapy to retain more control over both the pace at which issues are raised, and the opportunity to refrain from discussion of personal issues related to the interaction within the couple's relationship.

The purpose of therapeutic interaction, in couple or larger group situations, is to provide structure, support and guidance to enable people to modify their dysfunctional behaviour. However, the time spent in therapeutic sessions will invariably be a minute proportion of the time spent elsewhere, and so it is important that specific behavioural goals are set as steps towards overcoming the stated dysfunction. After the specific dysfunction has been defined, the purpose of the therapeutic interview then takes on the purpose of explaining a wide variety of sexual assignments which couples will be set for completion before subsequent sessions, and as a forum for the discussion of the successes and difficulties found in completing such assignments. The purpose of such assignments is to increase the couple's confidence and decrease the aversive component which has become associated with their sexual interactions, and is concordant with the views of Bandura (1969) noted earlier.

Such assignments are frequently seen initially as contrived and mechanical. It is important to explain the underlying rationale and to negotiate the final format of the activity with the couple, emphasising that it is essential to re-learn the practical aspects of lovemaking (which appears mechanical) in order that subsequent interactions may become more spontaneous and romantic.

Progress through such assignments is monitored in subsequent sessions. Whilst some couples find engaging in such activities to be rewarding and simple to establish, others report unwillingness to attempt such activities or find difficulty making time. Both types of response provide valuable clues for the therapist in assessing therapeutic progress, and often form the basis for discussion in subsequent sessions. For a comprehensive description of assignments, readers are again directed to the book by Jehu (1979).

A Case Study in the Treatment of Psychosexual Dysfunction

As the assignments set for couples vary as a function of the presenting condition, and will be modified dependent upon the progress through therapy, the following case study is provided as an example of a typical presenting condition which is amenable to behavioural change. For the sake of confidentiality a number of aspects from different cases are included.

Mr. and Mrs. A. The couple were aged 32 and 26 respectively at the time they presented with sexual difficulties, having been married for six years. Both were unemployed; Mr. A. because he found prospective employers tended not to offer him appointments once they saw him at interview, and Mrs. A. because of a congenital limb deformity.

Mr. A. suffered an incomplete lesion at the level of T10 four years earlier. He reported some pain at the lesion site and that he was able to drain urine using intermittent self catheterisation.

During the initial stages of the marriage they had some sexual difficulties because of the deformity to Mrs. A.'s legs; she found penetration painful at times, though both felt that this had not placed undue strain on the relationship. Mrs. A. reported that they had consummated the marriage though sexual activity at the present time was impossible because Mr. A. was unable to sustain an erection for more than a few seconds, and that even when this occurred attempts at penetration would result in immediate detumescence. Despite this, both reported that their marriage was very rewarding as they showed a great deal of affection to one another in other ways.

Preliminary investigations revealed no physiological basis for the difficulty, and NPT assessment results conducted over four consecutive nights showed erections lasting over 20 minutes and of sufficient rigidity for penetration on nine separate occasions.

It became clear during the first treatment session that although Mrs. A.'s limb deformity had made sexual intercourse slightly painful for her earlier in the marriage, subsequent surgery now means she experienced no pain although she felt her husband still held back. Mr. A. agreeed that this was true to some extent, but that his main reason for not attempting to penetrate at the present time was his inability to sustain his erection. Furthermore, Mr. A. commented that on occasions he may not be able to remain continent and this made him worry. Considerable time was therefore spent examining ways of avoiding accidents by careful monitoring of fluid intake and bladder drainage.

Following more detailed investigation, the partners were then seen separately. Such a procedure is often useful in such cases as it allows each to explore issues which they may find embarrassing raising in front of their partner.

In this particular case it became clear that Mr. and Mrs. A.'s previous sex life had not been particularly satisfying for either of them; for Mr. A. because of his feeling that his wife did not like to experiment and did not really like sex, and for Mrs. A. because she felt her husband did not spend long enough trying to arouse her and, as a consequence, she was often left feeling unsatisfied.

Their lack of understanding of one another's needs was discussed further when both were present. In order to examine the nature and importance of communication, they were asked to spend time at home either discussing or noting down the points they each liked and dislike about one another. Time was to be set aside on at least two occasions before the next session to discuss these issues in detail.

At this stage of treatment the couple were told not to attempt to have sexual intercourse under any circumstances. Whilst there is some disagreement (Clement and Schmidt 1983) as to whether a total ban on intercourse is of therapeutic value, it is considered desirable in problems of this kind because of the damaging results which further failure might have on their willingness to continue with therapy.

Mr. and Mrs. A. attended the second session two weeks later and reported that they had sat down and discussed their good and bad points and had spontaneously attempted to modify their behaviour accordingly. The session continued by exploring those areas in which compromises had been reached in the domestic situation, and then moved on to explore areas of sexual behaviour in which compromises might similarly be reached. It became clear that both partners' perceptions of the length of time Mr. A. spent providing sexual arousal for his wife were disparate. Mr. A. agreed that he probably did not spend much time providing stimulation for his wife but that once he began to become aroused he felt so anxious that the feeling might pass that he just wanted to get it over with. The rest of the session centred around an examination of the need for Mrs. A. to become aroused, both for her own benefit, but also in order to provide further stimulation to Mr. A. The session concluded by setting the couple the task of exploring one another's bodies to find those areas which each liked having stimulated.

At the start of session three the couple reported that they had been unable to attempt the exercises set because they had both begun attending an adult training centre and, upon their return home at night, had felt too tired. This course of action served as the basis of the discussion for this session with the therapist providing support to the couple for not having tried to force sexual interaction. It was further explained that to attempt sexual activity whilst tired would most likely result in failure or disappointment. A further session was set for two weeks later, and the couple were encouraged to attempt the exercises at the weekend when both felt more rested.

At the beginning of the fourth session, Mr. A. reported that they had spent a number of occasions engaging in touching exercises, and that on one occasion they had attempted sexual intercourse which had been satisfactory, which was confirmed by Mrs. A. Although Mr. A. found difficulty ejaculating as a result of his injury, he did still experience pleasurable sensation which culminated in a sensation similar to ejaculation. In questioning both partners further, it became clear that the episode of sexual intercourse had followed a particularly lengthy period of touching by Mr. A., with Mrs. A. reporting that she had been able to experience orgasm soon after penetration. Mr. A. similarly reported that he had been able to experience feelings of ejaculation and whilst this also had occurred very soon after penetration, he had at least been able to maintain the erection to allow penetration to take place.

It became clear during a brief session alone with Mr. A. that he could control the point at which he experienced the sensation of ejaculation when masturbating but during sexual intercourse he was worried about not being able to maintain the erection long enough to provide some satisfaction for his wife.

During the subsequent joint session it was decided that Mr. A. would provide stimulation in order to allow his wife to achieve orgasm and then spend time to increase her arousal prior to his wife providing stimulation for him. Both partners felt that this would reduce some of the worry Mr. A. felt concerning his wife's sexual enjoyment. They were also taught how to practise a technique in order that Mr. A. could begin to regain some control of his ability to maintain an erection, and reduce his fears concerning premature ejaculatory sensations.

The procedure entails the male being stimulated to the point just before involuntary ejaculation takes place. The male then has to get his partner to stop and allow his arousal to subside for approximately 30 seconds, and to repeat the procedure for a few times. The difficulty at first is learning the point at which to tell the partner to stop stimulating the penis, though after a number of attempts men are usually able to learn the process, and obtain some degree of competence in controlling the point at which they experience ejaculation, or the pleasurable feelings without physical ejaculation as in this particular case.

For those who have difficulty with this method, a squeeze technique is often recommended, which requires the partner to stop stimulation at the point immediately before ejaculation, and either person then squeezes the penis between finger and thumb at the base of the glans for approximately 10 seconds. This has the effect of reducing the reflex ejaculatory response and can also induce detumescence. If the latter occurs, it is usually possible to regain the erection within a few minutes, which often serves to increase the male's confidence in attaining erections.

During the following session, Mrs. A. reported that she was able to obtain orgasm during most of the occasions in which they attempted sexual activity. Mr. A. reported that he was able to maintain erections sufficient for penetration on most occasions and that the length of time they were maintained prior to ejaculation had also increased. They both stated that they still had times when things went wrong, but that they now felt more able to talk about why this might have occurred and not worry about it. Mr. A. reported that he had in fact produced urine during an occasion when he and his wife were practising the squeeze technique, but that they had simply been able to laugh it away. It also became clear, from the interaction between the couple, that whereas in the earlier sessions most of the communications had been directed towards the therapist, they now spent more time discussing issues raised by the therapist before they would make a joint response.

The following six sessions were all brief, as Mr. and Mrs. A. were experiencing no real difficulties during sexual activity. Assignments set gradually moved on from simultaneous caressing, to penetration without movement, and finally to penetration with movement and ejaculation. Therapy was concluded at the end of this series of sessions, with the understanding that if difficulties arose in the future, they were able to contact the therapist immediately.

Case Summary

Whilst the relationship was essentially rewarding for both partners, they had become able to predict one another's needs and so most activities were carried out with little discussion.

It is considered that therapy in this case, as in many others, was of value in overcoming their sexual difficulties as it re-established lines of communication. Those couples who report greatest benefit from therapy are those who make a comprehensive examination of one another's behaviour in the early sessions. Similarly, those who are more receptive and committed to the assignment exercises tend to pass through therapy more quickly, though given the high degree of individual variability in both the determinants and content of the presenting difficulty, there are no set guidelines for the number of sessions required. There are as yet no published data available from the present author's investigations but Cooper's (1969) assertions that those cases in which the partner co-operates in therapy respond significantly better would appear to have some validity. What is clear in most treatment sessions is that the therapist becomes somewhat redundant as couples increasingly resolve issues, raised in therapy, themselves.

Whatever the therapeutic strategy adopted by investigators for the treatment of psychosexual dysfunction, what remains clear is the need for more methodologically rigorous investigation. In no field is this more true than in the assessment of those factors associated with the development and maintenance of psychosexual dysfunction in people who have experienced spinal trauma. The use of objective assessment methods may be one way in which the efficacy of psychosexual counselling procedures may be established. There is some evidence available (Glass 1988) that day erection measurement pre- and post-treatment yields some useful findings, and the design of valid and reliable questionnaires for use at similar times, and at longer term follow-up, may prove useful.

References

Abrams K (1981) The impact on marriages of adult-onset paraplegia. Paraplegia 19: 253–259

Amelar R, Dubin L (1982) Sexual function and fertility in paraplegic males. Urology 20: 62–64

Bandura A (1969) Principles of behaviour modification. Holt, Rinehart and Winston, New York

Bardlach J, Anderson F (1979) Sexual therapy in rehabilitation. In: Murray R, Kijek J (eds) Current perspectives in rehabilitation nursing. Mosby, St Louis, pp 188–206

Barlow D, Becker J, Leitenberg H, Agras W (1970) A mechanical strain gauge for recording penile circumference change. J Appl Behav Anal 3: 73–76

Beard H, Sampson T (1981) Denial and objectivity in haemodialysis patients: adjustment by opposite mechanisms. In: Levy N (ed) Psychonephrology 1. Plenum, New York, pp 169–176

Beck J, Sakheim D, Barlow D (1983) Operating characteristics of the vaginal photoplethysmograph: some implications for its use. Arch Sex Behav 12: 43–58

Benson G, Lipshultz L, McConnell J (1983) Mechanisms of human erection, emission and ejaculation: current clinical concepts. In: Zorgniotti A (ed) Vasculogenic impotence. Thomas, Springfield, Illinois, pp 71–86

Bors E, Comarr A (1960) Neurological disturbance of sexual function. Urol Surv 10: 191–222

Brady J (1969) Brevital relaxation treatment of frigidity. Behav Res Ther 4: 71–77

Bregman S (1975) Sexuality and the spinal cord injured woman. Sister Kenny Institute, Minneapolis

Brindley G (1981) Reflex ejaculation under vibratory stimulation in paraplegic men. Paraplegia 19: 300–303

Brindley G (1984) The fertility of men with spinal injuries. Paraplegia 22: 237–245

Brindley G, Rushton D, Craggs M (1974) The pressure exerted by the external sphincter of the urethra when its motor nerve fibres are stimulated electrically. Br J Urol 46: 453–462

Clement V, Schmidt G (1983) The outcome of couple therapy for sexual dysfunctions using three different formats. J Sex Marital Ther 9: 67–79

Comarr A (1966) Observations on menstruation and pregnancy among female spinal cord injury patients. Paraplegia 3: 263–272

Conine T (1984) Sexual rehabilitation: the roles of allied health professionals. In: Kreuger D (ed) Rehabilitation psychology: a comprehensive textbook, Aspen System Corporation, Rockville, pp 124–158

Cooper A (1969) Disorders of sexual potency in the male: a clinical and statistical study of some factors related to short-term prognosis. Br J Psychiatry 115: 709–719

Fink S, Skipper J, Hallenbeck P (1969) Physical disability and problems in marriage. J Mar Fam 30: 64–74

Fisher C, Gross J, Zurch J (1965) Cycles of penile erection synchronous with dreaming (REM) sleep. Arch Gen Psychiatry 12: 29–45

Fisher C, Schiavi R, Edwards A (1976) Assessment of nocturnal REM erection in differential diagnosis of sexual impotence. Sleep Res 5: 42

Fisher C, Schiavi R, Edwards A (1979) Evaluations of nocturnal penile tumescence in the differential diagnosis of sexual impotence: a quantitative study. Sleep Res 6: 431–437

Fisher C, Cohen H, Shiavi R et al. (1983) Patterns of female sexual arousal during sleep and waking: vaginal thermo-conductance studies. Arch Sex Behav 12: 97–122

Fisher S (1973) The female orgasm. Basic Books, New York

Francois N, Lichtenberger J, Jouannet P, Desert J, Maury M (1980) Ejaculation by vibromassage in paraplegies: report of 50 cases with 7 pregnancies (in French). Ann Med Phys 23: 24–36

Franks C, Wilson G (eds) (1974) Annual review of behaviour therapy: theory and practice. Bruner/Mazel, New York

Freund K, Sedlacek F, Knob K (1965) A simple transducer for mechanical plethysmography of the male genitalia. J Exp Anal Behav 8: 169–170

Geer J, Morokoff P, Greenwood P (1974) Sexual arousal in women: the development of a measurement device for vaginal blood volume. Arch Sex Behav 3: 559–564

Glass C (1989) An investigation of some psychological factors of importance in the assessment and treatment of secondary impotence in dialysis and transplant patients. PhD thesis, University of Liverpool

Glass C, Fielding D, Evans C, Ashcroft J (1988) Factors related to sexual functioning in male patients undergoing haemodialysis and with kidney transplants. Arch Sex Behav 16: 189–207

Gutmann L (1964) The married life of paraplegics and tetraplegics. Paraplegia 2: 182–188

Jehu D (1979) Sexual dysfunction: a behavioural approach to causation, assessment and treatment. Wiley, New York

Kaplan H (1974) The new sex therapy: active treatment of sexual dysfunctions. Bruner/Mazel, New York

Karacan I (1969) A simple and inexpensive transducer for quantitative measurement of penile erection during sleep. Behav Res Methodol Inst 1: 251–252

Karacan I (1970) Clinical value of nocturnal erection in the prognosis and diagnosis of impotence. Med Asp Hum Sex 4: 27–34

Karacan I, Catesby Ware J, Dervent B et al. (1978) Impotence and blood pressure in the flaccid penis: relationship to nocturnal penile tumescence. Sleep 1: 125–132

Kilmann P (1978) The treatment of female orgasmic dysfunction: a methodological review of the literature since 1970. J Sex Marital Ther 4: 155–176

Kinsey A, Pomeroy W, Martin C, Gebhard P (1953) Sexual behavior in the human female. Saunders, Philadelphia

Lamid S (1985) Nocturnal penile tumescence studies in spinal cord injured males. Paraplegia 23: 26–31

LoPiccolo L, Heiman J (1978) Sexual assessment and history interview. In: LoPiccolo J, LoPiccolo L (eds) Handbook of sex therapy. Plenum, New York, pp 233–238

Marshall P, Surridge D, Delva N (1981) The role of nocturnal penile tumescence in differentiating between organic and psychogenic impotence – the first stage of validation. Arch Sex Behav 20: 1–10

Masters W, Johnson V (1966) Human sexual response. Little Brown, Boston

Masters W, Johnson V (1970) Human sexual inadequacy. Little Brown, Boston

McCarthy B (1973) A modification of Masters and Johnson's sex therapy model in a clinical setting. Psychother Theor Res Prac 10: 290–293

Money J (1960) Phantom orgasm in the dreams of paraplegic men and women. Arch Gen Psychiatry 3: 373–382

Nagler B (1950) Psychiatric aspects of cord injury. Am J Psychiatry 107: 49–56

Ohlmeyer P, Brilmeyer H, Hullstrung H (1944) Periodische Vorgauge in Schlaf. Pfluegers Arch Ges Physiol 248: 559–560

Polack J, Gu J, Mina S, Bloom S (1981) Vipergic nerves in the penis. Lancet 2: 217–219

Ryan J (1961) Dreams of paraplegics. Arch Gen Psychiatry 5: 94

Schuler M (1982) Sexual counselling for the spinal cord injured: a review of five programmes. J Sex Marital Ther 8: 241–252

Shambaugh P, Hampers P, Bailey G, Snyder D, Merril J (1967) Haemodialysis in the home: emotional impact on the spouse. Trans Am Soc Artif Intern Organs 13: 41–45

Sha'ked A, Flynn R (1978) Normative sexual behaviour and the person with a disability: training of rehabilitation personnel. J Rehabil 44: 30–36

Trieschmann R (ed) (1980) Spinal cord injuries: psychological, social and vocational adjustment. Pergamon Press, New York

Virag R, Virag H, Lajujie M (1985) A new device for measuring penile rigidity. Urology 25: 80–81

Wagner G (1981) Erection: physiology and endocrinology. In: Wagner G, Green R (eds) Impotence: physiological, psychological and surgical diagnosis and treatment. Plenum, New York, pp 25–36

Wasserman M, Pollak C, Spielman A, Weitzman E (1980) The differential diagnosis of impotence:

the measurement of nocturnal penile tumescence. J Am Med Assoc 243: 2038–2042

Weiss H (1972) The physiology of human penile erection. Ann Intern Med 76: 793–799

Wolpe J (1958) Psychotherapy by reciprocal inhibition. Stanford University Press, California

Wolpin M (1969) Guided imagining to reduce avoidance behaviour. Psychother Theor Res Prac 6: 122–125

Zuckerman M (1971) Physiological measurement of sexual arousal in the human. Psychol Bull 75: 297–329

Chapter 8

Anaesthesia

J.W.H. Watt

Introduction

The physiological disability of a patient with a spinal cord injury presents the anaesthetist with a number of different and substantial problems. It is useful for the surgeon to have some insight into these problems as they may influence both the choice and conduct of anaesthesia and the outcome. The wide spectrum of neurological disability and concurrent problems demand that the anaesthesia for a specific procedure be tailored to the patient in order to provide satisfactory operating conditions and to minimise the overall risk to the patient.

Following acute spinal cord injury (ASCI) with a neurological deficit there is a period of so-called spinal shock during which time the spinal motor neurones below the level of the lesion remain inexcitable. The spinal shock resolves gradually over a few weeks and the rate of recovery varies considerably between cases; between the autonomic and somatic systems; and in a longitudinal sense, from the sacral to cervical segments. Flaccid paralysis persists in those segments with a lower motor neurone lesion but, commonly, monosynaptic reflexes return with spastic paralysis below the level of the neurological insult.

Though the great majority of urological operations are undertaken in patients who have reached a state of neurological stability, which may be called chronic spinal cord injury (CSCI), surgery may be required for patients with ASCI. For instance, bilateral ureteric obstruction secondary to pelvic fractures and haematomata may require decompression, or a seriously disrupted bladder may require repair. The discussion must therefore firstly consider anaesthesia for patients with ASCI, drawing attention to features which are specific to that phase in addition to features which persist into the chronic stable state.

Anaesthesia and Acute Spinal Cord Injury

Cardiovascular System

When a patient with ASCI presents for surgery the anaesthetist will wish to confirm the neurological level in order to interpret the concomitant cardiovascular changes. Lesions at or above T4 may be associated with a sinus rhythm of between 40 and 50 beats per minute and occasionally with varying degrees of atrioventricular block. If anticholinergic drugs such as atropine are given regularly simply to elevate the pulse rate to normal levels, there is a risk of toxicity with confusion and restlessness quite apart from aggravation of ileus, unpleasant dryness of the mouth and interference with the recovery of bladder function during intermittent catheterisation. Nevertheless, atropine should always be available since patients with lesions above the sympathetic outflow may develop severe vagal slowing and sinus arrest in association with hypoxaemia and certain stimuli such as tracheal suctioning.

Spinal shock is commonly associated with systemic hypotension and a systolic pressure of 90–100 mmHg due to peripheral vasodilatation but this does not usually call for aggressive corrective measures in the absence of severe atheromatous disease. If a bradycardia is present atropine may well usefully improve the blood pressure. Alternatively, the nebulisation of a beta-2 agonist drug such as salbutamol, which can be given for mucous clearance and bronchodilatation, will result in a modest elevation of the pulse rate and blood pressure. Parenteral beta-2 agonists are to be avoided in ASCI since they have been known to cause profound vasodilatation and cardiovascular collapse.

Before assuming a neurological cause for hypotension, haemorrhagic hypotension must be considered. A low central venous pressure (CVP) measurement may point to hypovolaemia but conversely its ability to warn of overtransfusion is limited because of the poor correlation between the CVP in ASCI and left atrial pressure. The latter correlates more closely with the risk of pulmonary oedema. It is not uncommon that patients are overtransfused in the attempt to raise the systemic blood pressure in the face of a profound vasodilatation and this is a common cause of pulmonary oedema in ASCI. A patient without overt pulmonary oedema who undergoes anaesthesia and intermittent positive pressure ventilation (IPPV) can develop florid pulmonary oedema on discontinuation of the IPPV. The propensity to pulmonary oedema is greater in patients with loss of the cardiac sympathetic innervation and impairment of cardiac contractility. The measurable surge in catecholamines immediately after ASCI is not sustained and so the genesis of the pulmonary oedema is not a massive shift of fluid as in acute head injury. Another predisposing factor is the hypoalbuminaemia which can develop quite rapidly in the presence of ileus and sepsis. The anaesthetist will be guided in the assessment of pulmonary oedema either invasively by pulmonary artery catherisation, or more simply by clinical features, arterial oxygenation, fluid balance and the chest X-ray.

If cardiac inotropic drugs are required, low-dose dopamine has the advantage in ASCI of increasing heart rate and arterial blood pressure as compared with dobutamine, which may decrease arterial blood pressure (Butterworth et al. 1987). It is well recognised that in chronic spinal cord injury there is an increased sensitivity to vasopressors but it is not clear how soon such denervation sensitivity appears.

Respiratory System

Acute respiratory insufficiency after ASCI can be quite insidious and hypoxaemia is extremely common following injuries at all spinal levels. Patients with lesions around the third to fifth cervical segmental level may develop diaphragmatic fatigue a day or two after ASCI and slide into respiratory failure and cardiorespiratory arrest. At this neurological level patients may also suffer from sleep apnoea. Comparing high with low thoracic lesions there is a progressive loss of inspiratory capacity and effort, and of expiratory effort and force of coughing so that a patient with a lesion at a thoracic level one or two with normal use of the arms has virtually as much respiratory disability as the patient with a fifth cervical lesion. On top of such a neurological loss, pulmonary pathology may precipitate respiratory failure. Such pulmonary pathology encompasses pulmonary oedema, gastric aspiration, water inhalation, trauma to the rib cage and associated pleural pathology, sputum retention with atelectasis as well as pneumonia. Narcotic analgesics must be used with care in the vulnerable patient during this acute period and chest physiotherapy provided to treat and prevent respiratory complications.

The neurological level after ASCI will often ascend one or two segments in the days following injury and such a borderline patient may fail to breathe adequately after surgery and anaesthesia and require postoperative IPPV. When prolonged respiratory assistance is anticipated a tracheostomy should be considered.

Conduct of Anaesthesia

Control of the Airway

Surgery in the acute phase is usually carried out under general anaesthesia because of possible interventions required in a physiologically unstable patient and because the patient is unlikely to have much insight into his medical condition. Nevertheless, the induction of anaesthesia presents considerable hazards in addition to the cardiorespiratory vulnerabilities already described.

The patient may have gastric dilatation or gastric bleeding if not treated prophylactically with antacids and usually the patient would need a nasogastric tube to reduce the risk of gastric aspiration. After a cervical injury the neck may be maintained in extension causing difficulties in laryngoscopy and endotracheal intubation or even in access if halo traction is applied. On occasions the larynx must first be intubated under cover of local anaesthesia before proceeding to general anaesthesia but either way ample time may be required for the induction of anaesthesia.

In other circumstances the anaesthetist would consider using the rapidly acting muscle relaxant suxamethonium to secure the airway but after both upper and lower motor neurone lesions the administration of suxamethonium causes a massive potassium efflux from skeletal muscle with records of hyperkalaemia as high as 13 mmol/l. The period of sensitivity starts from 48 hours after injury (Gronert and Theye 1975) and persists in non-progressive cases at least for 12 months (Cooperman 1970). In progressive conditions this sensitivity remains. Cardiac arrest following the use of suxamethonium in ASCI is well documented in the literature.

Anaesthesia Maintenance

Patients with ASCI subjected to general anaesthesia commonly respond with a fall in blood pressure below the preoperative value due to the effects of volatile agents as well as the induction agents, and also due to positive pressure ventilation. Such a response is exaggerated in the presence of toxaemia from lower respiratory or urinary tract infection so that inotropic support may be required. Blood loss would be dealt with in the usual way bearing in mind the twin risks of hypotension and pulmonary oedema.

Other problems for the anaesthetist include maintenance of temperature, care of the skin and maintenance of the vertebral alignment intraoperatively and during transfer.

Anaesthesia and Chronic Spinal Cord Injury

Preoperative Evaluation

In contrast with the acute patient, anaesthesia for the patient with chronic spinal cord injury (CSCI) is generally less hazardous. Nevertheless, despite their adaptation for activities of daily living they do have reductions in the physiological reserve with certain specific vulnerabilities. The conduct of the anaesthesia is closely determined by the findings at the time of preoperative assessment.

The anaesthetist will make a neurological examination to confirm the motor and sensory level of the lesion, whether the latter is complete or incomplete, and whether the paralysis is spastic or flaccid. Somatic hyperreflexia in patients with lesions above the T6 level correlates with the propensity to autonomic hyperreflexia in response to visceral distension or other stimuli such as the surgeon's knife. Above T6 the visceral vascular bed participates in reflex vasoconstriction and the resulting shift in blood volume and reduction in vascular capacitance produce severe hypertension which if unmodified may progress to cerebral haemorrhage, convulsions or cardiac failure. The hypertension is characteristically accompanied by bradycardia, mydriasis and sweating within a minute of an appropriate stimulus. This together with reflex spasms in the legs and abdomen necessitates some form of anaesthesia in many operative procedures.

Patients with incomplete lesions may have sympathetic preservation which may be assessed whilst the patient performs a Valsalva manoeuvre, most easily done by attempting to maintain a pressure of 40 mmHg on an aneroid gauge for 15 seconds (McLeod and Tuck 1987). Records of the resting heart rate would suggest sympathetic preservation if the rate had exceeded 120 beats per minute. Tachycardia below this rate simply suggests withdrawal of parasympathetic tone.

At rest, the systolic blood pressure bears a linear relation to the neurological level, changing by 2 mmHg per segment (Frankel et al. 1972). The blood pressure is usually lower in the sitting position. The renin-angiotensin system compensates for postural falls in blood pressure (Mathias and Frankel 1983) but it remains the case that profound hypotension may follow abrupt postural changes such as may occur during the positioning of patients for surgery.

Since essential hypertension is not common in this group of patients, the finding of systolic hypertension may be indicative of renal disease. Creatinine production is reduced in the paralysed patient and the Cockcroft and Gault formula for the estimation of creatinine clearance from the serum creatinine (cr) should be corrected by a factor of 0.8 and 0.6 for paraplegic and tetraplegic patients respectively (Mirahmadi et al. 1983). Thus if the body weight is in kg and the serum creatinine in μmol/l the formula simplifies to:

$$kg \times \frac{(146 - age)}{cr}$$

for paraplegics, and

$$kg \times \frac{(146 - age)}{cr} \times 0.72$$

for tetraplegic patients.

The importance to the anaesthetist of impaired renal function resides in the impaired clearance of peripherally acting muscle relaxants, antibiotics, and baclofen; accompanying anaemia, hyperkalaemia or acidosis and in the intraoperative maintenance of renal perfusion and function. If amyloid is implicated the possibility of adrenal infiltration and insufficiency would need to be considered.

The assessment of respiratory function begins with inspection for features such as scoliosis, or tracheostomy scar which may forewarn of a potential subclinical subglottic stenosis. Observation will also reveal the extent of paralysis of the respiratory musculature in cases with paradoxical movement of the chest on respiration, and the vital capacity measured at the bedside may be reduced by over 50% from the predicted value. Furthermore, in patients dependent upon the diaphragm, the vital capacity shows a further fall of 15% in moving from the supine to sitting position. Some patients may only manage a vital capacity of one litre even when supine. They may have chronic basal atelectasis and are at risk from postoperative chest infection which is poorly tolerated as is abdominal distension. An increase of tracheobronchial secretions is hazardous for the tetraplegic who may rely on assisted coughing. In the extreme, profuse secretions immediately on awakening from general anaesthesia may asphyxiate the patient; lesser degrees of sputum retention will predispose to lower respiratory tract infection. Prophylactic antibiotics are indicated in some of these patients together with preoperative physiotherapy and training in the technique of positive pressure breathing and the use of incentive spirometers.

A more general review of the patient will assess other features such as cervical rigidity, ankylosing spondylitis, and chronic flexion contractures which may present difficulties during positioning of the patient on the operating table and even, in some cases, for surgical access. The skin condition should be noted with regard to vulnerable pressure sites. Patients with CSCI and chronic infections who undergo anaesthesia are especially prone to acute systemic hypotension upon induction of anaesthesia and preliminary fluid loading is necessary. Whilst the history and examination are being carried out an assessment of the patient's mental state is made so that the anaesthetist can decide how best to advise the patient if there is a choice between general and local anaesthesia.

Regional Anaesthesia

Excepting patients with flaccid paralysis, some form of anaesthesia is necessary to control the reflexes during endoscopic surgery, for which topical anaesthesia alone is inadequate. Spinal anaesthesia is well suited to much endoscopic surgery although a proportion of patients will ask for general anaesthesia and other patients have local factors which preclude a lumbar puncture. Flexion of the spine may be difficult but antispasmodic premedication helps overcome spastic lordosis. This author considers there to be a relative contraindication to spinal anaesthesia in patients with incomplete lesions or without a neurological diagnosis in case of apparent inexplicable deterioration in the neurological status postoperatively.

Spinal anaesthesia does not disturb the respiratory system of the tetraplegic patient and for that reason alone is safer. It provides a tranquil operating field with some reduction in operative bleeding in relation to the fall in systemic blood pressure and it avoids the coughing and straining sometimes associated with recovery from general anaesthesia, which may suddenly increase bleeding risking a catheter blockage. In comparison with a lumbar epidural anaesthetic, a spinal is both quicker technically and in its onset of action and, in addition, gives more reliable reflex protection considering that an epidural anaesthetic is usually based upon a catheter technique with adjustment of the dosage according to the sensory level attained on testing.

Despite its relative safety, spinal anaesthesia is not without its hazards. The main one is systemic hypotension, for example, on lowering the legs from lithotomy position though this may also occur during general anaesthesia and in other groups of patients. It might be expected that hypotension resulting from spinal anaesthesia per se would be less of a problem in the patient with CSCI with, in effect, a sympathectomy. The author has reviewed the records from the last 5 years of 150 patients having urological surgery, 44 of whom had spinal anaesthesia. A number of these patients had repeated procedures with up to 5 separate spinals in one case.

There was no consistent relationship between the intraoperative blood pressure and either the neurological level or the immediate preoperative blood pressure, although there was a tendency for the blood pressure response to the spinal in any individual to be similar from one occasion to the next. A greater mass of local anaesthetic or a higher spread did increase the incidence of hypotension. Some patients had no fall in blood pressure whereas for example a C5 "complete" tetraplegic patient had a fall of blood pressure from 120/65 to 85/40 mmHg within 5 minutes. Despite the fact that the resting noradrenaline levels are lower than normal (Debarge et al. 1974), it may be that a lesion proximal to the spinal sympathetic interneurones does not abolish a degree of tone in the sympathetic vasculature which is then susceptible to the local anaesthetic block.

A less well recognised complication of spinal anaesthesia is the appearance of bradycardia which may progress to asystole. Schonwald et al. (1981) recorded an incidence of bradycardia of 8% occurring unpredictably and as late as 30 minutes after induction, confirming the need for electrocardiographic monitoring in all cases. The bradycardia can be due to a blockade of the sympathetic outflow to the heart at T4 in a paraplegic patient. Bradycardia can also develop as a chronotropic response to a low filling pressure in the great veins and right atrium due, in turn, either to the anaesthesia or blood loss (Greene 1981). The opposing reflex from the carotid sinus to maintain the pulse and blood pressure depends upon an intact efferent limb of the arc. A prompt autotransfusion on raising the legs briskly or the Trendelenberg position increases the heart rate quicker than atropine can do. Nevertheless, both atropine and a selected vasopressor are always to hand and in some cases are given prophylactically.

Endoscopic surgery can also be carried out under cover of caudal epidural anaesthesia since a suitable dose of local anaesthetic will abolish the local parasympathetic reflexes whilst preserving the tone of the sympathetically innervated smooth muscle of the pelvic vasculature with a reduction in bleeding. The unreliability of caudal anaesthesia in achieving a sensory block may be less important in the CSCI patient but, on the other hand, an inadequate block may manifest itself by systemic hypertension or priapism. The stimulus of bladder distension may in fact require the block to extend to T10 to prevent reflex hypertension at which level there would then also be blockade of the pelvic sympathetic vasculature. In practice, a low caudal anaesthetic may be combined with a general anaesthetic using the latter to control the systemic blood pressure.

General Anaesthesia

Inhalational anaesthesia may be administered by face mask with spontaneous respiration for minor procedures in patients with powerful diaphragmatic respiration despite intercostal paralysis. Otherwise, tracheal intubation and relaxant anaesthesia is selected for the greater control the anaesthetist has over the patient's physiology. The latter technique ensures better gas exchange and reduces the tendency to atelectasis which the tetraplegic patient is ill-equipped to correct postoperatively. Airway instrumentation may engender secretions which could be troublesome during the recovery period but a small dose of atropine will minimise this problem in addition to giving protection against reflex bradycardias as a result of manoeuvres such as airway suctioning in the presence of hypoxaemia.

General anaesthesia and controlled ventilation is the preferred technique for percutaneous lithotripsy because the procedure is rather long for a conscious patient to tolerate in the semi-prone position with restricted respiration and it prevents untoward patient movement at crucial moments. Furthermore, the management of the complications of this procedure is easier if general anaesthesia is administered from the outset. These potential complications have been reviewed by Peterson and colleagues (1985) and include the absorption of large volumes of irrigating fluids systemically to cause hyponatraemia and, rarely, disseminated intravascular coagulation, or into the pleural space to cause hydropneumothorax. Intraoperative monitoring of pulmonary compliance and the use of an oesophageal stethoscope permits early detection of such complications and, if necessary, arterial oxygenation, acidity and haematocrit may be checked.

Relaxant anaesthesia should also reduce the risk of unexpected coughing or straining during endoscopy compared with inhalational anaesthesia and spontaneous respiration. Nevertheless, because it is often possible to maintain a lighter plane of anaesthesia in patients with loss of sensation there is the chance of sudden movement with a lightening of the depth of anaesthesia if the neuromuscular block is not maintained.

The suppression of autonomic reflexes under general anaesthesia may require high concentrations of volatile agents which are provided more safely with controlled ventilation and prevention of hypercapnia and minimisation of myocardial depression. Given in this way, an agent such as halothane is as effective as a regional technique in blocking hypertensive responses at the cost of a deep anaesthetic and a slow recovery which is less convenient for a short procedure.

Despite this propensity to reflex hypertension, systemic hypotension poses a greater threat to CSCI patients undergoing general anaesthesia. This occurs particularly upon induction of anaesthesia but also in response to the volatile agents and positive pressure ventilation though fluid loading will often suffice to contain the effect.

General anaesthesia is inferior to regional anaesthesia with regard to the control of reflex priapism. Even high concentrations of volatile agents may be relatively ineffective. Ketamine which has been advocated for the relief of priapism is itself an anaesthetic and analgesic and has complex interactions with catecholamines, including a reduction of re-uptake at peripheral adrenergic endings. However, its efficacy in priapism may depend upon intact corticospinal pathways. The author has found it to be effective in a patient with an incomplete paraplegia but ineffective in two patients with complete lesions. By contrast, doses of a ganglion-blocking agent such as 5 mg of trimetaphan, insufficient to cause significant hypotension, can effectively control the priapism.

The problem of temperature control is similar whatever anaesthetic is used though there is additional heat loss under general anaesthesia caused by inhalation of dry gases unless a humifier is used and it is generally necessary to take measures to minimise heat loss. Oesophageal thermometry is advocated for procedures such as percutaneous lithotripsy which may make the patient hypothermic or, alternatively, bacteraemic with a temperature high enough to warrant exclusion of the condition of malignant hyperpyrexia. Usually the anaesthetist administers antibiotics intraoperatively according to the unit policy.

Postoperative Care

Patients hypothermic after general anaesthesia should have oxygen therapy until well recovered and some patients may require specific respiratory therapy postoperatively in co-operation with the physiotherapist. Systemic analgesics are often not required but may help control severe autonomic hyperreflexia. Otherwise, chlorpromazine or phenoxybenzamine may be used to control postoperative hypertension.

Patients who take the antispasmodics diazepam or baclofen are at risk of developing convulsions if the drugs are abruptly discontinued postoperatively because of ileus. Baclofen is not readily available for parenteral use but diazepam may be used as an alternative until oral intake is resumed.

Conclusion

The patient with either acute or chronic spinal cord injury requiring urological surgery presents a number of specific problems to the anaesthetist. These cover every system but in particular affect the cardiovascular, respiratory and neuromuscular systems. An understanding of the pathophysiology is essential in planning the most appropriate anaesthetic technique and in anticipating abnormal responses to procedures. Because many anaesthetists do not commonly encounter such patients, good liaison between the urologist, the spinal injury specialist and the anaesthetist enables the last to evaluate the anaesthetic problems and to help plan a safe operation.

References

Butterworth JF, Austin JC, Johnson MD et al. (1987) Effect of total spinal anesthesia on arterial and venous responses to dopamine and dobutamine. Anesth Analg 66: 209–214

Cooperman LH (1970) Succinyl-induced hyperkalemia in neuromuscular disease. JAMA 213: 1867–1871

Debarge O, Christensen NJ, Corbett JL, Eidelman BH, Frankel HL, Mathias CJ (1974). Plasma catecholamines in tetraplegics. Paraplegia 12: 44–49

Frankel HL, Michaelis LS, Golding DR, Beral V (1972) The blood pressure in paraplegia. Paraplegia 10: 193–198

Greene NM (1981) Physiology of spinal anaesthesia, 3rd edn. Williams & Wilkins, London

Gronert GA, Theye RA (1975) Pathophysiology of hyperkalemia induced by succinylcholine. Anesthesiology 43: 89–99

Mathias CJ, Frankel HL (1983) Clinical manifestations of malfunctioning sympathetic mechanisms in tetraplegia. J Auton Nerv Syst 7: 303–311

Mc Leod JG Tuck RR (1987) Disorders of the autonomic nervous system: Part 2. Investigation and treatment. Ann Neurol 21: 519–529

Mirahmadi MK, Byrne C, Barton C, Perera N, Gordon S, Vaziri ND (1983) Prediction of creatinine clearance from serum creatinine in spinal injury patients. Paraplegia 21: 23–29

Peterson GN, Krieger JN, Glauber DT (1985) Anaesthetic experience with percutaneous lithotripsy. Anaesthesist 40: 460–464

Schonwald G, Fish KJ, Perkash I (1981) Cardiovascular complications during anesthesia in chronic spinal cord injured patients. Anesthesiology 55: 550–558

References

Chapter 9

Innovations and Future Possibilities

E.P. Arnold

Introduction

The standard of care and the quality of life for patients with spinal cord injuries have improved enormously in the last 40–50 years, and along with these has come a very significant reduction in mortality.

Specialised units caring for the needs of the spinal cord injured are now established in most countries. Prior to that patients often languished in the corner of busy wards inexperienced in the special needs of the paralysed person. With the development of these units has come the rapid growth of the new speciality of Rehabilitation Medicine with its valuable holistic approach, and the expansion of biomedical engineering expertise, which can allow some assistance in environmental control for patients with even very high levels of injury.

There have been improvements in the standard of nursing care and the avoidance of pressure sores, and in physiotherapy and occupational therapy; there has been an expansion in the range of antibiotics available and in their efficacy; and extracorporeal lithotripsy of renal stones, common in spinal cord injury patients due to infection and skeletal calcium absorption from immobilisation, has been an enormous advance.

Advances in the orthopaedic care of cervical injuries mean that some patients can be mobilised early in "halo" traction, and avoid several weeks of dependency and often despondency, lying in bed with skull traction. This can have a considerable impact on the patient's outlook and ability to adjust to his or her disability.

Tendon transfers in those with C7 injuries may produce "key grip" movements which could enable the patient to do intermittent self catheterisation, or even be able to manage bladder emptying with sacral anterior root stimulation.

Standing wheelchairs, which may be electrically or hydraulically driven, enable occasional eye level contact with others and this can be a great morale booster for someone getting accustomed to being talked down to.

Electrical stimulation of "walking" is being more widely used. Some devices employ external electrodes placed over the femoral and peroneal nerves to lock the hip and the knee straight while the patient swings the pelvis forward and walks on straight pegs. Other methods employ implanted electrodes to do the same. Sophistication has led to some being computer driven so that the surface electromyography signals characteristic of upper torso movements during walking, are picked up from the erector spinae muscles, and translate to functional electrical stimulation of the appropriate leg to straighten it and generate supported gait. (Mizrahi et al. 1985). Many Units are now using the Parawalker.

The relationship between lower urinary tract dysfunction and upper tract damage has been stressed by many authors since Talbot and Bunts (1949) drew attention to it. Bors (1954) noted a renal mortality of 2% in those with balanced bladder function in contrast to 31% with unsatisfactory bladder function. Webb et al. (1984) further reduced mortality to 0.5% in 406 patients followed for 15 years.

Expansion in the availablity of urodynamics in the last 20 years has led to a greater understanding of the significance of lower urinary tract dysfunction and its role in the pathogenesis of upper tract damage. In turn this has meant better and clearer indications for intervention in order to prevent damage from obstruction or vesico-ureteric reflux (Arnold et al. 1984).

Regular intermittent self catheterisation has become a widely accepted method of ensuring complete bladder emptying with an acceptably low rate of complications including clinical urinary tract infection. Many patients, even those with reflex bladders, have become continent and appliance free with or without the assistance of medication.

More recent urological innovations include the use of electronic means to control voiding and continence, erections and ejaculation. Future developments will see these improve, become more computerised, and perhaps become noninvasive. New research may open the possibility for nerve regeneration and grafting to reduce the neurological deficit after a spinal cord injury.

Electronic "Control" of Autonomic Functions

A major aspect of the devastation caused to a person by a spinal cord injury is the lack of ability to control the body's autonomic functions, especially of micturition, defaecation and continence, and also of erection and ejaculation. A considerable amount of work has been done in the last two decades in seeking electrical and other means of regaining some control. Notable successes in the clinical field of sacral anterior root electrostimulation have been achieved by Brindley and his team in London, and by Tanagho and Schmidt in San Francisco.

Historical Review

Continence

On theoretical grounds continence might be gained by increasing the striated sphincter tone by chronic electrical stimulation, or by reducing the excitability of the micturition reflex, or by increasing the use of the functional bladder capacity.

Increasing Outlet Resistance

Implanted Sphincter Electrodes. Electrodes implanted on the urethral sphincter or anal sphincter were described by Caldwell et al. in 1963 and 1965; they showed that both anal and urinary incontinence could be controlled in some cases. An interesting observation was that after several months of use some patients no longer needed to use the electrical stimulation to keep continent.

Bazeed et al. (1982) produced experimental evidence that chronic electrical stimulation can increase the bulk of the external sphincter, and suggested that it might also increase the proportion of fatigue-resistant type 2 muscle fibres.

Surface Stimulation. Anal plug electrodes were used by Hopkinson and Lightwood (1967) with some success in about half their patients. Brindley et al. (1974) described a modification of the anal plug through which more efficient stimulation of motor fibres could be achieved. Alexander et al. (1970) described their use of a vaginal pessary electrode for continuous stimulation of the adjacent urethral sphincter. Fall et al. (1978) used a similar device. However, many patients refused to persist and did not like wearing such devices, so they are not widely used today.

Sacral Anterior Root Stimulation (SARS). Another approach has been chronic stimulation using sacral anterior root stimulators to close the urethra, aiming to choose stimulation parameters that excite somatic efferents to contract the external sphincter, but that do not stimulate the parasympathetic fibres supplying the bladder. This has not been a particularly useful approach to date.

Dampening Reflex Detrusor Contractions

By electrical stimulation of pudendal nerve afferents Sundin et al. (1974) were able to produce detrusor inhibition in the cat. Intravesical electrical stimulation of the bladder using a special electrocatheter was shown to cause reduction in the excitability of the micturition reflex by Katona and Berenyi (1975). Merrill (1979) used the Mentor Continaid for transrectal stimulation and found an increase in detrusor reflex threshold in 4/20 cases. These four patients achieved continence but leaking resumed on ceasing stimulation. These stimulators may act also by increasing outlet muscle contraction and improving the outlet resistance.

Madersbacher et al. (1982) used similar techniques for patients with spinal cord injury. More recently Vodusek et al. (1986) used stimulation of the pudendal nerve afferents to demonstrate reflex inhibition in patients with spinal cord injuries. It is possible that antidromic stimulation of the sacral anterior roots might alter the excitability of the reflex in some way (Bradley 1971). Reflex contractions should be abolished by cutting posterior roots but might be suppressed due to nerve root damage at the time of nerve root implant surgery in those whose posterior roots have not been deliberately cut. However, damage due to the latter cause usually recovers and the reflex returns.

Facilitating Full Use of the Functional Bladder Capacity

With uninhibited reflex contractions the bladder rarely if ever empties to completion because of dyssynergic contractions of the striated muscle of the pelvic floor and urethra, or because the detrusor does not continue to contract until the bladder is completely empty. About 70% of such patients are dry on intermittent self catheterisation programmes, some with the aid of anticholinergic medication (Cass et al. 1984; Arnold et al. 1989). A similar proportion of patients using sacral anterior root stimulation of voiding 4–6 times a day are dry probably for the same reasons (Brindley et al. 1986a).

Electromicturition

The principle of a radio-transmitter applied to the skin over a buried receiver was described first by Chaffey and Light in 1934 when they used it to stimulate a monkey's brain. It was subsequently used for urological stimulation by Bradley et al. in 1962. It avoided some of the problems of infection and size that had previously complicated transcutaneous wires or buried pacemakers (Hageman 1966; Hald et al. 1966; Alexander and Rowan 1968). Movement often led to fractured cables; infection was common; the electrodes tended to erode into the bladder; and current spread led to pain and stimulation of the outlet resistance at the time of voiding.

Attempts to gain control over the bladder and urethra electronically, have developed along the following three main lines.

Direct Stimulation of the Bladder or Pelvic Nerves

Electrodes implanted onto the bladder wall were first used by Boyce at al. in 1964, and several authors since, but have not been widely used. Theoretically, they might have a place in those with cauda equina lesions as the implant could then stimulate intact post-ganglionic fibres even if the pre-ganglionic fibres have been destroyed by the spinal cord lesion. However, experimentally Brindley (1984a) was unable to stimulate the bladder directly in a baboon which had undergone a division of those anterior roots known to supply the bladder a week earlier.

Unipolar carbon fibre electrodes implanted on the bladder wall were used recently by Petersen et al. (1986) who found that these electrodes were better tolerated than metal ones, and that there was less current spread with the unipolar than with previously used bipolar electrodes. They were hopeful such a device could be useful in flaccid denervation where SARS was not applicable.

Because the pelvic nerves are in the form of a plexus, defining a specific nerve around which to place an electrode is impossible. Moreover, the pelvic plexus does not tolerate the strength of electrical stimulation required and nerve damage may ensue (Tanagho and Schmidt 1988).

Stimulation of the Conus Medullaris

This method was developed by Nashold et al. (1972), Grimes et al. (1973) and Jonas and Tanagho (1975). The first group reported its use in five paraplegics of whom three had a long-term success. The in-depth electrodes were positioned in the intermedio-lateral gray columns of the cord adjacent to the descending reticulo-spinal pathways, at S1 level or lower.

Sacral Anterior Root Stimulation (SARS)

Habib (1967) reported the use of SARS in animals and in humans, and Brindley (1973, 1977) reported his experience in baboons and in several papers since then on its clinical use.

The San Francisco group have produced detailed studies of preliminary research, and the subsequent development for clinical use of SARS with the electrodes placed extradurally, and combined with selective pudendal neurectomy to reduce any concomitant contraction of the sphincter at the time of bladder stimulation (Tanagho and Schmidt 1988). This aims to allow continuous stimulation and achieve continuous flow. Although successful in achieving continence in all their patients, satisfactory voiding occurred in only 8 of 24 patients.

A similar technique was described by Talalla et al. (1986) and also used extradural electrodes.

The Problem of Stimulation-Induced Detrusor-Sphincter Dyssynergia

SARS of S2, 3 and 4 causes contraction of the pelvic floor and urethra as well as contraction of the detrusor muscle. To overcome this unwanted outflow resistance, Brindley (1973) explored intermittent stimulation in a baboon model. Later he reported (Brindley 1977) on the clinical use of bursts of stimulation with voiding occurring between bursts. The striated muscle at the outlet contracts rapidly and the detrusor more slowly. In the gap between bursts, the outlet relaxes rapidly while the slower detrusor is still contracting, resulting in post-stimulation voiding (Fig. 9.1).

With the Brindley technique, usually within the first 6–9 months after the operation, the stimulus parameters have to be reduced as the inevitable neuropraxia of the operation recovers. Should detrusor pressures prove to be too high, they can be reduced by adjustment of the stimulus parameters within the control box, usually by reducing the stimulus frequency.

External sphincterotomy has been used for a few patients in whom the spastic contraction of the pelvic floor and urethral sphincter has precluded voiding and resulted in high pressures. This is at the expense of a somewhat reduced incidence of continence between electro-voidings. Similarly, this also applies to the patient who has had a sphincterotomy before the Brindley stimulator has been inserted. Further, the pressures are only high at the time of stimulated voiding as long as the posterior roots have been cut, and pressures at other times are quite flat. Hence the upper urinary tracts have not been damaged by continuous use of the implant, in some cases now for over 15 years.

With the Bladder Pacemaker developed in San Francisco by Tanagho and Schmidt, the roots of S3 are approached extradurally. Other roots are tested and,

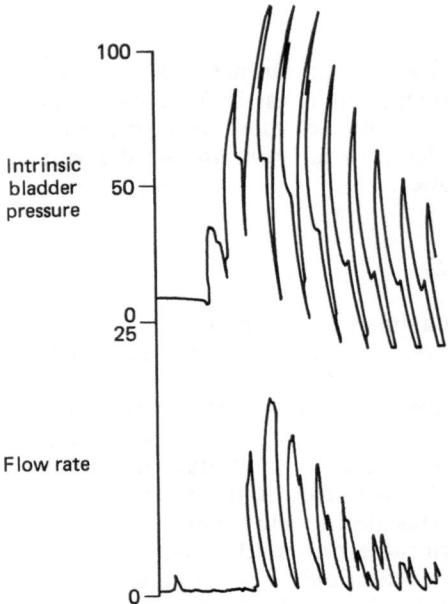

Figure 9.1 Urodynamic recording of detrusor pressure and flow rate demonstrating lag between stimulation and voiding.

if they produce additional contractions of the detrusor, then an electrode is placed around them too. To overcome any residual concomitant striated muscle contraction of the urethra, a selective division of urethral nerve fibres travelling with the pudendal nerve is undertaken, usually 4–6 weeks after the pacemaker implantation (Schmidt 1988).

SARS: the Present Situation

The Brindley-Finetech Stimulator is the most widely used type at this time and the most successful in achieving good bladder emptying as well as continence.

Operative Details

At laminectomy via an intradural approach, the anterior roots of S2, S3 and S4 are identified on each side from anatomical location of the cauda equina and the exit of the nerves. The exact identity of each nerve is confirmed by electrical stimulation and then by observing muscular activity in the pelvic floor and distal limb muscles, and recording bladder and rectal pressure responses. The anterior roots are separated from the posterior. Sometimes it is impossible to separate the anterior and posterior roots of S4, in which case they are included together. Occasionally the S5 nerve is intimately associated with the S4 and is then incorporated with S4 in that electrode booklet. A similar dissection is performed on each side. The anterior roots of S2, S3 and S4, plus or minus the combined motor and sensory nerve of S5, are positioned in the slots of the booklet electrode as illustrated in Fig. 9.2a. From it, cables are led subcutaneously to a radio receiver buried in the subcutaneous tissues of the anterolateral chest wall. Within the buried receiver block there are three radio receivers with different frequency tunings, one for each pair of nerve roots (Fig. 9.2b).

Following operation when voiding is desired, a palm-sized radio-transmitter is applied to the skin overlying the receiver so that its three coils for the trapped roots, are immediately under those same coils of the transmitter. The latter is connected by a cable to the signal generator control box which allows adjustment of strength, frequency, shape and timing of the electrostimulation. The parameters are adjusted to achieve optimal detrusor contraction and the most efficient emptying.

When bladder emptying is desired the patient positions himself or herself either on a toilet or using a receptacle to collect urine. The transmitter is held over the receiver, the orientation of which can be felt under the skin, so that the stimulating coils are over the appropriate receiver coils and the control box is switched on.

The nerve supply of the detrusor is the same as for the sphincter. With stimulation of the anterior roots the detrusor smooth muscle contracts slowly while the striated muscle of the sphincter contracts rapidly. Hence stimulation is made in bursts so that while the detrusor is contracting strongly the stimulation stops and

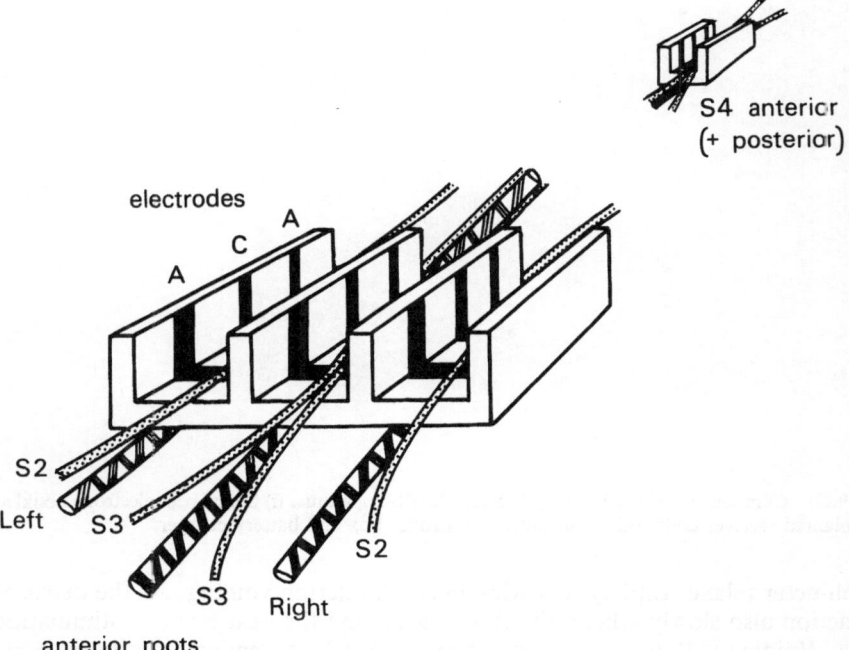

Figure 9.2.a Location of nerve rootlets within the stimulator electrode.

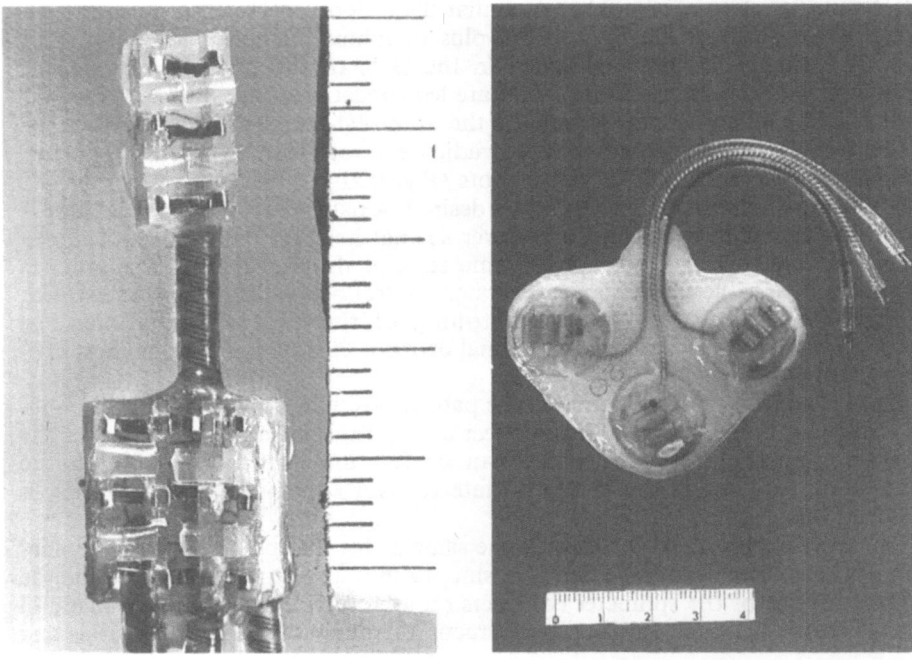

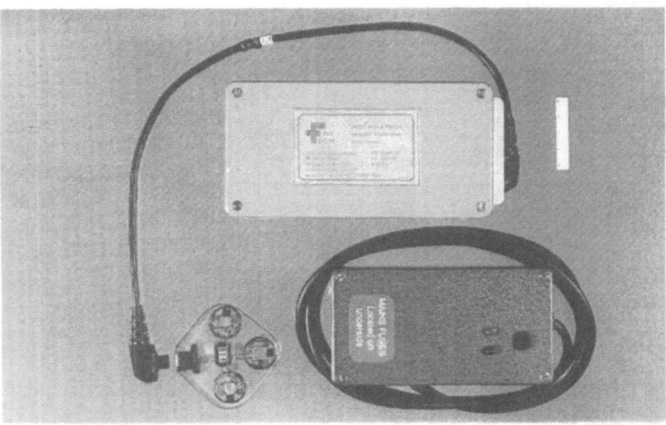

Figure 9.2b Components of the Brindley-Finetech SARS apparatus. (i) Spinal root electrode booklet. (ii) Implanted receiver coils. (iii) Transmitter, controller box and battery charger.

the sphincter relaxes rapidly, allowing post-stimulation voiding. As the detrusor contraction also slowly relaxes the flow ceases, and the next burst of stimulation arrives. Voiding is thus intermittent. (See Fig. 9.1.) The patient continues to use the stimulator until flow ceases. Residual urine is usually as low as 0–50 ml.

By adjustments made within the control box, a burst is programmed to continue until an adequate detrusor pressure response has occurred, and to re-start at the time when the detrusor pressure induced by the last contraction is falling. Voiding pressures can be controlled by adjusting the stimulating parameters within the control box. High pressures can be reduced best by shortening the time of each burst or, alternatively, by reducing frequency or strength.

For some who have had the outlet resistance reduced by an external sphincterotomy, the electrostimulation can be continuous, and will produce a continuous flow. This is often possible in females without the above procedures having been done, because of the lower urethral resistance. However, posterior rhizotomies are now advocated in females as they enhance continence by abolishing reflex detrusor contractions (Madersbacher et al. 1988).

Division of Posterior Roots

This is advised now for both the Brindley and the Tanagho Bladder Pacemaker types of sacral anterior root stimulator. Division of posterior roots should abolish or minimise reflex detrusor contractions. This has the advantage of producing a larger functional bladder capacity and an improved rate of continence between stimulated voidings. It can abolish the pain associated with electrostimulation in those with incomplete lesions.

The disadvantage of dividing posterior roots in the male is that it will abolish reflex erections; however, such erections are not always satisfactory for sexual function and in any case the disadvantage may be partly offset by the ability electrically to drive erections by continuous stimulation of the S2 anterior roots in about 30% of men. Even should that not be possible there remain other methods of achieving erection by intracavernous injections of active drugs such as papaverine. If S3 and S4 posterior roots are cut and S2 spared, this might preserve erections while still increasing the functional bladder capacity.

Division of posterior roots also has the disadvantage of denervating skin, abolishing its neurotrophic effects and perhaps predisposing to pressure area injury.

If posterior roots are to be cut then these effects must be fully discussed with the patient. If the roots are not cut, then it is still possible to do it later or to complete the deafferenting in those in whom it has been selective and has not produced the desired result in reducing the excitability of the micturition reflex.

Other Aspects of Surgical Technique

The approach via an extended laminectomy of L3 to S2 advocated by Brindley has not resulted in significant problems with scoliosis or spinal deformity, but should be avoided in children under 16 years. If intrathecal fibrosis is extensive a modified electrode can be placed lower down extradurally. As yet it is not known whether the extradural approach is associated with any less risk of damage to the nerve roots than the intradural method.

Case Selection

The patient should be neurologically stable and should be psychologically motivated and adjusted to the fact of his or her disability. In our experience this usually takes 12–18 months. The efferent limb of the sacral micturition reflex needs to be intact. This can be demonstrated if uninhibited detrusor contractions are observed during filling cystometry. However, if cystometry shows reduced compliance but no definite contractions, their presence should be sought by electrostimulation of the pelvic plexus with a glove-mounted transrectal electrode before an implant is contemplated (Brindley 1981).

Use of the device should increase the patient's independence. This implies that upper limb function must be sufficiently preserved to allow transfer to a toilet or to hold the urinal whilst using the radiotransmitter. Hence, relatively few quadriplegics stand to gain much from the device.

Notwithstanding the above, most of those with complete lesions of the thoracic cord who have adequate hand function are suitable. Caution is required for those with an incomplete lesion as electrical stimulation might result in pain. This too can be tested preoperatively by transrectal stimulation of the pelvic plexus. As discussed above, division of posterior roots can abolish such pain.

Previous outlet surgery including sphincterotomy may compromise the achievement of continence in some patients, but is not a contraindication to the placement of a sacral anterior root stimulator. Females have more to gain than males as there is no suitable external collecting device available for women, and the results of SARS are good for both voiding and continence (Madersbacher et al. 1988).

Autonomic dysreflexia is not a contraindication provided that the posterior roots are divided at the time of the implant.

Results

The Brindley-Finetech apparatus has been used in a number of centres throughout the UK, in New Zealand, Australia, France, Austria, and some other areas. Approximately 250 implants have been performed at the time of writing.

Benefits to be expected include the ability to void by electrical stimulation down to a negligible residual urine, with the consequent reduction in incidence of urinary infections. Most patients become continent and appliance-free. Many find improved bowel function and, for about 30% of the men, it is possible to achieve electrical stimulation of erection.

Electromicturition

Among the first 50 cases reported by Brindley et al. (1986), 44 (88%) were able to achieve good detrusor pressures and efficient voiding. Of the 6 implants not then in use, 3 stopped because of associated pain (dorsal roots not cut), 1 had nerve root damage, 1 anomalous roots and 1 electronic component failure awaiting repair.

In our small group of 7 patients operated in Christchurch, 6 have a functioning implant and one does not, probably due to anomalous nerve roots, as previously discussed (Arnold et al. 1986). Of the 6 in use the residual urine is between 0 and 30 ml, while the peak flow rate has been 18–25 ml/second (Fig. 9.3.)

Urinary Infections

Of the patients who have had a problem with frequent infections before the use of electromicturition 31 of 38 (80%) have found a much decreased incidence postoperatively. This is due to the reduced residual urine and the complete emptying of the bladder 5–6 times a day (Brindley et al. 1986).

Continence

In those who have had the posterior roots divided, the occurrence of reflex uninhibited detrusor contractions is minimised as the reflex arc is no longer intact. As a result they have an increased functional capacity, without involuntary detrusor contractions.

Of the 44 patients using the Brindley controller, 30 were continent day and night (68%), and a furthur 5 were continent by night but not totally so by day. Of the women 9 out of 10 were reliably dry and appliance-free (Brindley et al. 1986; Madersbacher et al. 1988). Even in patients in whom the posterior roots were not divided, continence has been achieved in most. This has meant an appliance-free status has been reached unless the person is unsure when he or she will be able to reach a toilet to use the stimulator. Taking of alcohol and the related diuresis has made continence less reliable in some. Similarly, in those who

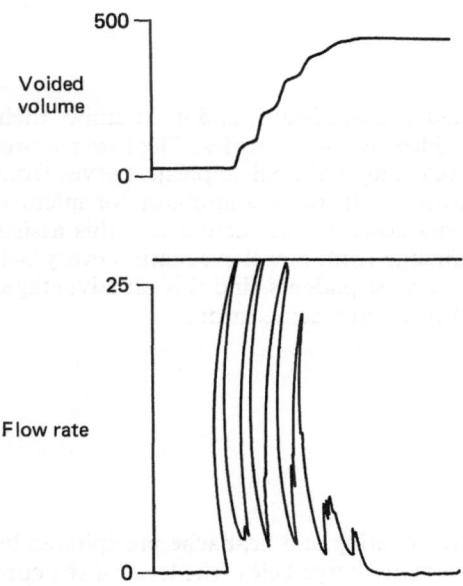

Figure 9.3 Peak flow rates at electromicturition.

develop a urinary infection this may temporarily compromise continence.

Continence has been of great benefit to the patients particularly at night when most can manage 8–10 hours or more of appliance-free sleep. This certainly enhances dignity and self image and the potential for sexuality expression unimpeded by an external collecting device, or by a wet bed.

Electro-erection

Stimulation of the S2 anterior nerve root usually produces an erection in the male. With the Brindley sacral anterior root stimulator programmed for strong continuous stimulation of S2, erection can be produced in some men and may last as long as the stimulus is continued. Among the first 50 patients reported by Brindley et al. (1986) there were 38 men and erections were possible by electrical stimulation in 26. For some with initial success, the quality of the erection deteriorated with time, for reasons not yet clarified.

Spontaneous reflex erections may be lost in the placement of the electrodes around the sacral roots due to neuropraxia of either afferent or efferent nerve roots, and patients need to be warned of this. Of course, if posterior nerve roots are deliberately cut as described above in the current technique, then reflex erections will definitely be abolished. However, the advantage of cutting posterior roots often outweighs this, as in many cases erections can be electrically stimulated, and for those for whom this is not possible erection can be achieved by intracavernosal injections of vasoactive drugs.

Using stimulation parameters set for electromicturition, a minor degree of penile engorgement may occur in some males but this has not been sufficient to interfere with micturition. Headache and a raised blood pressure from autonomic dysreflexia may occur sometimes with electrical stimulation of erection.

Bowel Function

Spinal cord injury patients are constipated almost always, and most empty their bowels by digital evacuation sometimes aided by suppositories. The lower bowel is supplied with parasympathetic fibres reaching it via pelvic plexus nerves from the dominant S4 root. Many patients using the Brindley stimulator for micturition find it will bring the colonic contents down to the rectum and this assists digital evacuation. Its use may mean a change from bowel evacuation every two days to the need to do this every day, but most patients find this an advantage. A few patients can achieve implant-driven electro-defaecation.

Complications

Autonomic Dysreflexia

This refers to reflex hypertension, diffuse sweating and headache precipitated by vascular spasm caused by mass sympathetic discharge below the level of the cord lesion in response to any other activity below the lesion. Notable in this regard is autonomic activity such as bladder contractions, retention or catheterisation, bowel evacuation or enemata, or somatic activity such as a pressure area or fracture. The hypertension is sensed by baroceptors on the aortic arch and carotid sinus and relayed to the vasomotor centre, which tries to reduce blood pressure by vasodilatation of vessels in skin of segments above the level of the lesion with which it is still in contact. Sweating occurs along with this. The condition occurs in about 30% of patients using electromicturition but usually improves within the first year of use.

Electrical stimulation of micturition or ejaculation can cause such dysreflexia as discussed above.

Upper Urinary Tract Damage

Vesico-ureteric reflux can be demonstrated in about 10% of patients after a spinal cord injury. After prolonged use of the sacral anterior root stimulator in the first 50 cases, Brindley et al. (1986a) reported two cases of caliceal dilatation. In some cases reflux had ceased following use of the implant, but in no case had the degree of reflux deteriotated. One new case of reflux has been reported, but is not of a degree indicating clinical significance.

SARS produces a type of dyssynergic voiding, with the potential for high pressures at peaks of stimulation; however, the height of stimulated pressure can be reduced by adjustments within the control box. Further, if posterior roots have been cut, the pressures are high only at the time of stimulated voiding; pressures at other times are quite flat. Hence the upper tracts have not been damaged by continuous use of these implants, in some cases now for over 15 years.

Nerve Root Damage

In the early cases, posterior root damage is known to have occurred in 4 of the 13 with incomplete lesions of the cord, who had tactile sensation preoperatively and then lost it. Posterior root damage does not recover (Brindley et al. 1986a).

Anterior root damage occurred in 23 of the first 50 cases. In most this was transient and had recovered by the end of the first year, in many completely. Over half of these cases were able to use implant-driven micturition despite the known damage (Brindley et al. 1986a). No patient has experienced nerve degeneration as a result of stimulation for voiding or for continence. One patient in England died by suicide after three years continuous use of SARS; at autopsy there was no significant damage or scarring of the roots.

Cerebrospinal Fluid Leak

In the earlier cases, cerebrospinal fluid leaked around the cables emerging from the dura and presented as a swelling around the buried receiver block. This occurred in 14 of the 50 and required a surgical re-exploration in order to cure it. The others settled conservatively. It has been much less of a problem since the routine use of the improved grommet to gain a seal around the cables emerging from the dura.

Implant Infections

To avoid implant infections prophylactic antibiotics are given. The cables and receiver block and electrode mounts are all constructed using antibiotic-impregnated silicone rubber (Rushton et al. 1989).

Implant Failures

There were 13 problems representing technical failures in 11 patients in the first 50 cases. These were 5 tunnel connectors, 4 fractured cables, 2 plug and socket connectors, and 3 receiver block failures. This covered 154 patient years of experience. Most of these were repaired subsequently. We have had two patients with fractured cables, one in the midline posteriorly too close to the electrode to be repaired by rejoining the cables. He had the same roots placed in electrodes extradurally lower down in the spinal canal and the posterior roots were cut at the re-operation. He now voids very satisfactorily and is continent. The patients with cable fractures have been vigorous sportsmen playing wheelchair basketball and it is thought that the cables fractured when repeatedly stressed against the back of the wheelchair.

When an implant fails for whatever reason, providing the posterior roots have not been divided, reflex bladder emptying will resume as before the operation. The patient then can revert to the use of clean intermittent self catheterisation (CISC) or an external collecting device. If the posterior roots have been cut, the bladder will be flaccid and then would require CISC, or some other means of assisted emptying.

Summary

The main benefit to patients in having the stimulator is in the vastly improved self image, and the continence which is achieved in most cases, so that collecting devices or catheters are not required. Although some technical failures have occurred in the accumulated experience with using this implant, these have been able to be repaired in most cases quite simply by replacing the receiver block or the cable connections. The intradural electrodes have been quite reliable and have not needed to be replaced.

Whilst electro-erection has been possible in some, it is not reliably achieved by the procedure and at this stage should not be considered an indication for implant.

SARS is a significant step forward for a limited number of patients with spinal cord injuries, as it will allow a continent device-free interval between episodes of stimulated voiding, and with reduced incidence of urinary infections because of a negligible residual urine. It improves a patient's self image and dignity as well as independence.

Sexual Function

The need for love including physical proximity and sexual expression is universal, and is very strong in the young which is the group most often afflicted with traumatic spinal cord injury. Infertility in the spinal cord injured male relates to erections which, if achievable, are not necessarily sustainable for function, and to ejaculatory failure in many. Of those who do ejaculate, sperm quality is often inferior.

Reflex erections rely mainly on sacral parasympathetic outflow and should occur so long as the sacral segments of the cord and the cauda equina remain intact. Psychogenic erections, however, are not necessarily lost in patients with damage below L2 and above S2. It has been suggested that the descending spinal tracts responsible may have access to sympathetic erectile pathways (Bors and Comarr 1960; Brindley 1984b). Psychogenic erections occur in the absence of sympathetic input as after a retroperitoneal lymph node dissection. The role of the sympathetic nervous system in patients with parasympathetic decentralisation remains to be clarified. Ejaculation requires that T12–L2 and the sympathetic outflow be intact.

Erection

Reflex erections adequate for coitus are possible in some patients after spinal cord injury, but for some are unsustained and unsatisfactory. For these, there are the options of intracavernous injections of vasoactive drugs such as papaverine. The dose must be adjusted down, as those with neuropathic problems have been found unusually sensitive to medication and there is a risk of priapism. Patients who have a sacral anterior root stimulator may be able to achieve electro-erections as discussed above.

In some centres, prosthetic penile implants have been used for sexual purposes or to assist in the wearing and application of external collecting devices (Rossier and Fam 1983). There is a small risk of ulceration and erosion due to unnoticed trauma.

Obtaining Semen

Some patients after spinal cord injury can ejaculate at the time of coitus. For those who cannot, two artificial techniques are available and both can be used at home without much difficulty. However obtained, the semen then requires artificial insemination, for example using a fine Tom Cat catheter (Brindley 1981).

Electro-ejaculation

Ejaculation is not dependent on erection. It is essentially a sympathetic efferent excitation centred on T12–L2, with fibres traversing the hypogastric plexus before reaching the pelvic plexus. Stimulation of the hypogastric plexus results in seminal emission but not the clonic movements of the pelvic floor and anal sphincters and the ischio-cavernosus muscles associated with normal orgasm.

Electro-ejaculation can be performed by transrectal stimulation of the pelvic plexus (Brindley 1981). S1–L2 somatic function can be tested by scratching the sole of the foot which should produce reflex hip flexion, and stimulation of the obturator nerve which should produce hip adduction. If both tests are positive, electrical stimulation of emission should be possible. The technique may produce pain in incomplete cord injuries. General anaesthesia with muscle relaxants can then be used to obtain semen.

Initial studies by Brindley showed that electro-ejaculation in some patients produced fluid containing sperm, in others none was produced but the next voided urine contained more than 5 million sperm, and in still others no sperm were produced at all. In Christchurch during transrectal electrostimulation, a catheter with a small balloon is pulled back against the bladder neck to prevent retrograde passage of semen into the bladder. Autonomic hyperreflexia can occur with electrostimulation and blood pressure should be checked regularly throughout.

The quality of semen is often indifferent in spinal cord injury patients particularly in relation to poor motility. This has led to the practice in some centres of offering to undertake electro-ejaculation and storage of semen from the first week or so after injury. Obtaining semen by electrical stimulation at home is not as easy as with the vibrator, and not all spouses wish to learn the technique. Where the vibrator is not successful, it is a reasonable alternative.

Vibro-ejaculation

Vibrators of specific frequency, applied to the glans will often produce an emission in approximately 70% of men (Beretta et al. 1989). Commercially available vibrators with a range of 2.5 mm and a frequency of 60–100 Hz have been found to be the most effective. They are expensive but produce a semen of better quality than with electro-ejaculation. It carries a risk of autonomic dysreflexia which is particularly marked in lesions above T5. Blood pressure should be recorded during stimulation. It will not function in complete conus or cauda equina lesions. Time since injury did not influence outcome.

The semen is generally of poor quality with both of these methods, but is better after vibro-ejaculation than with electrical stimulation, which also tends to produce retrograde ejaculation; urine is a poor medium for preservation of semen.

Electro-ejaculation was successful in 3 of 4 men with levels of injury below T12, and with 5 of 8 above T11. Vibro-ejaculation was successful in none of 9 with levels of injury below T12, but was successful in 18 of 28 above T11 (Bielby and Keogh 1989).

Hypogastric Plexus Stimulators

This has been tried by Brindley (1986), and involved electrodes around the plexus at the level of the aortic bifurcation. He reported two patients, both of whom produced semen but their partners did not become pregnant.

Vas Cannulation and Sperm Reservoirs

Where vibration and electrical stimulation have failed, Brindley et al. (1986b) reported on 5 paraplegic men in whom the vas was cannulated and the silastic tube connected to an implanted silicone reservoir in the anterior abdominal wall. After sexual stimulation the reservoir could be punctured and semen obtained. One pregnancy was achieved and one implant had to be removed because of infection.

Artificial Spermatoceles

Alloplastic spermatoceles have not been particularly successful but Marman et al. (1984) used an expanded polytetrafluorethylene and were able to obtain sperm but they were all non-motile.

Female Sexuality

Sexuality in women with spinal cord injuries has been largely disregarded in the literature, but a good review was produced recently by Berard (1989).

Amenorrhoea is common for 3–9 months after a spinal cord injury. Thereafter, contraception is probably safest using an IUD rather than hormonal methods with their added risks of thrombogenesis and hypertension. During pregnancy, care is required due to the risk of autonomic hyperreflexia, particularly in those with high lesions. There is also an added risk of urinary infections, constipation, thrombogenesis and osteoporosis.

Delivery management should be considered according to the level of injury. For those with lesions above T10, labour and vaginal delivery should be possible although the risk of autonomic hyperreflexia is there, especially if the lesion is above T6. Assistance may be required as expulsive forces may be ineffective.

For those with lesions T10–T12, the uterus may not be areflexic, but caesarean section may be needed. Those with lesions below T12 and absent sensation are liable to perineal tears.

Pregnancy and successful vaginal delivery were reported in two women using sacral anterior root stimulators for voiding and continence without any untoward side-effects (Arnold et al. 1986; Nanninga et al. 1988).

Future Possibilities

Nerve Root Reconstruction

Experimental work has paved the way for the future possibility that the damaged cord could be bypassed by anastomosing nerve roots from just above the cord damage to those emerging from the damaged cord or just below it. Carlsson and Sundin (1980) reported two paraplegic patients with fractures of T12 and L1, managed by open reduction and stabilisation. At that operation the T12 mixed roots were divided 2–3 cm distal to the ganglion, and re-routed intradurally. The S2 and S3 dorsal and ventral roots were divided close to the cord, and T12 anastomosed to these using a tubularised silastic filter. At 12 months one patient had a return of bladder sensation and could void.

Vorstman et al. (1987) have shown it is feasible to divide intercostal nerves and to re-route the proximal end to reach the sacral roots intradurally for anastomosis. Experimentally in cats they performed a direct anastomosis between adjacent roots, and in other studies used a short segment of nerve graft to bridge the gap. Subsequent histological and electrical testing confirmed return of function in some (Vorstman et al. 1986).

Cord Regeneration?

It is known from animal experiments and human observations that a spinal cord transection does not regenerate, but some interesting experimental work is continuing.

Excision of a segment of dorsal columns in the cat and replacement by a graft of a segment of peripheral nerve was followed by axon growth from dorsal root origin and from axons within the central nervous system (Wardrope and Wilson 1986). They produced no evidence of functional connections.

In another study on rats, hemicordotomy was followed by sacrifice at 4–12 weeks. Controls had developed a depressed scar at the site, and the cord caudal to the transection had degenerated. In the study group of animals immediately after the transection, the gap was filled with a minced segment of peripheral nerve. The study showed not only regeneration across the gap but also that the caudal segment appeared intact, although the nerve fibres in the segment showed signs of degeneration. They conjectured that the Schwann cells of the grafted tissue might help in the repair and perhaps act as a trophic agent (Khalili and Hamash 1988).

It is difficult at this stage to see the relevance of these studies to any possible application in the human as the exact extent of the neurological lesion is often unclear at the time of a spinal cord injury. In the future this may be clarified by more sophisticated electrophysiological studies including cortical transit times and sensory- and motor-evoked potentials and latencies, aided by newer magnetic induction methods which are less painful than electrical stimulation.

Summary

As in many areas of medicine exciting advances in technology have improved immensely the quality as well as the length of life that can be expected by patients even with severe and grossly disabling conditions such as spinal cord injury. Perhaps the greatest problem facing us will be in matching what is technically possible with what is realistically affordable by the person and by society.

References

Alexander S, Rowan D (1968) Electrical control of urinary incontinence by radio implant: a report of 14 patients. Br J Surg 55: 358–364

Alexander S, Rowan D, Millar W, Scott R (1970) Treatment of urinary incontinence by electric pessary. Br J Urol 42: 184–190

Arnold EP, Fukui J, Anthony A, Utley WLF (1984) Bladder function following spinal cord injury: a urodynamic analysis of the outcome. Br J Urol: 56: 172–177

Arnold EP, Gowland SP, MacFarlane MR, Bean AR, Utley WLF (1986) Sacral anterior root stimulation of the bladder in paraplegics. Br J Urol 58: 319–324

Arnold EP, Anthony A, Henderson S, Schousboe M (1989) Intermittent self catheterisation and a catheter storage tube: a review of experience in a neuropathic bladder. In: Proceedings of the Urological Society of Australasia, Melbourne

Bazeed MA, Thuroff JW, Schmidt RA, Wiggin DW, Tanagho EA (1982) Effect of chronic electrostimulation of sacral roots on the striated urethral sphincter. J Urol 128: 1357–1362

Berard E JJ (1989) The sexuality of spinal cord injured women: physiology and pathophysiology. A review. Paraplegia 27: 99–112

Beretta G, Chelo E, Zanollo A (1989) Reproductive aspects in spinal cord injured males. Paraplegia 27: 113–118

Bielby JA, Keogh EJ (1989) Spinal cord injuries and anejaculation. Paraplegia 27: 152

Bors E (1954) Bladder disturbances in the management of patients with injury to the spinal cord. J Int Coll Surg Bulletin 21: 513

Bors E, Comarr AE (1960) Neurological disturbances of sexual function with special reference to 529 patients with spinal cord injuries. Urol Surv 10: 191–222

Boyce WH, Latham JE, Hunt LD (1964) Research related to the development of an artificial electrical stimulator for the paralysed human bladder. J Urol 91: 41–51

Bradley WE, Wittmers LE, Chou SN, French SA (1962) Use of a radio transmitter receiver unit for the treatment of the neurogenic bladder. A preliminary report. J Neurosurg 19: 782–786

Bradley WE, Timms GW, Chou SN (1971) A decade of experience with electronic stimulation of the micturition reflex. Urol Int 26: 283

Brindley GS (1973) Emptying the bladder by stimulating sacral ventral roots. J Physiol 237: 15–16

Brindley GS (1977) An implant to empty the bladder or close the urethra. J Neurol Neurosurg Psychiatry 40: 358–369

Brindley GS (1981) Electroejaculation: its technique, neurological implications and uses. J Neurol Neurosurg Psychiatry 44: 9–18

Brindley GS (1984a) Electrical stimulation in vesico-urethral dysfunction. In: Mundy AR, Stephenson TP, Wein AJ (eds) Urodynamics: principles, practice and applications. Churchill Livingstone, Edinburgh, pp 381–388

Brindley GS (1984b). The fertility of men with spinal cord injuries. Paraplegia 22: 237–245

Brindley GS, Rushton DN, Craggs MD (1974) The pressure exerted by the external sphincter of the urethra when its motor fibres are stimulated electrically. Br J Urol 46: 453–462

Brindley GS, Polkey CE, Rushton DN, Cardozo L (1986a) Sacral anterior root stimulation for bladder control in paraplegics – the first 50 cases. J Neurol Neurosurg Psychiatry 49: 1104–1114

Brindley GS, Scott GI, Hendry WF (1986b) Vas cannulation with implanted sperm reservoirs for obstructive azoospermia or ejaculatory failure. Br J Urol 58: 721–723

Caldwell K PS (1963) The electrical control of sphincter incontinence. Lancet 2: 174–175

Caldwell K PS, Flack FC, Broad AF (1965) Urinary incontinence following spinal cord injury treated by electronic implant. Lancet 1: 846–847

Carlsson CA, Sundin T (1980) Reconstruction of afferent and efferent nervous pathways to the urinary bladder in two paraplegic patients. Spine 5: 37–41

Cass AS, Luxenberg M, Gleich P, Johnson CF, Hagen S (1984) Clean intermittent catheterisation in the management of the neurogenic bladder in children. J Urol 132: 526–528

Chaffee EL, Light RU (1934) Radiofrequency link to stimulate the monkey brain. Yale Biol Med 7: 83–128

Fall M, Erlandson BE, Nilson EA, Sundin T (1978) Longterm intravaginal electrical stimulation in urge and stress incontinence. Scand J Urol Nephrol [Suppl] 44: 55–60

Grimes JH, Nashold BS, Currie DP (1973) Chronic electrical stimulation of the paraplegic bladder. J Urol 109: 242–245

Habib IN (1967) Experience and recent contributions in sacral nerve stimulation of voiding in both human and animal. Br J Urol 39: 73–83

Hageman J, Flanigan S, Harvard BM, Glenn W WL (1966) Electromicturition by radio frequency stimulation. Surg Gynecol Obstet 123: 807–811

Hald T, Agrawal G, Kantrowitz A (1966) Studies in stimulation of the bladder and its motor nerves. Surgery 60: 848–866

Hopkinson BR, Lightwood R (1967) Electrical treatment of incontinence. Br J Surg 54: 802–805

Jonas U, Tanagho EA (1975) Studies on the feasibility of urinary bladder evacuation by direct spinal cord stimulation. 2. Post-stimulation voiding – a way to overcome outflow resistance. Invest Urol 13: 151–153

Katona F, Berenyi M (1975) Intravesical transurethral electrotherapy in myelomeningocele patients. Acta Paediatr Acad Sci Hung 16: 363–374

Khalili AH, Hamash OH (1988) Spinal cord regeneration: new experimental approach. Paraplegia 26: 310–316

Madersbacher H, Paver W, Reiner E, Hetzch H, Spanudakis S (1982) Rehabilitation of micturition in patients with incomplete spinal cord lesions by transurethral electrostimulation of the bladder. Eur Urol 8: 111–116

Madersbacher H, Fischer J, Ebner A (1988) Anterior sacral anterior root stimulator (Brindley): experience especially in women with neurogenic urinary incontinence. Neurourol Urodyn 7: 593–601

Marman JL, DeBenedictus TJ, Praiss DE (1984) Clinical experience with an artificial spermatocele. Andrology 5: 304–311

Merrill DC (1979) The treatment of detrusor incontinence by electrical stimulation. J Urol 122: 515–517

Mizrahi J, Braun Z, Najenson T, Graupe D (1985) Quantitative weight bearing and gait evaluation of paraplegics using functional electrical stimulation. Med Biol Eng Comput 23: 101–107

Nanninga JB, Einhorn C, Deppe F (1988) The effect of sacral nerve stimulation for bladder control during pregnancy: a case report. J Urol 139: 121–122

Nashold BS, Friedman H, Glenn JF, Grimes JH, Barry WF, Avery R (1972) Electromicturition in paraplegia: implantation of a spinal neuroprosthesis. Arch Surg 104: 195–202

Petersen T, Christiansen P, Nielsen B, et al. (1986) Experimental electrical stimulation of the bladder using a new device. Urol Res 14: 53–56

Rossier AB, Fam BA (1983) Indications and results of semirigid penile prostheses in spinal cord injury patients: long-term follow up. J Urol 131: 59–62

Rushton DN, Brindley GS, Polkey CE, Browning GV (1989) Implant infections and antibiotic-impregnated silicone rubber coating. J Neurol Neurosurg Psychiatry 52: 223–229

Schmidt RA (1988) Applications of neurostimulation in urology. Neurourol Urodyn 7: 585–592

Sundin T, Carlsson CA, Kock NG (1974) Detrusor inhibition induced from mechanical stimulation of the anal region and from electrical stimulation of pudendal nerve afferents. Invest Urol 11: 374–378

Talalla A, Bloom JW, Nguyen Q (1986) Successful intraspinal extradural sacral nerve stimulator of bladder emptying in a victim of traumatic spinal cord transection. Neurosurgery 19: 955–961

Talbot HS, Bunts RC (1949) Late renal changes in paraplegia: hydronephrosis due to vesico-ureteric reflux. J Urol 61: 870–882

Tanagho EA, Schmidt RA (1988) Electrical stimulation in the clinical management of the neurogenic bladder. J Urol 140: 1331–1339

Vodusek DB, Light JK, Libby JM (1986) Detrusor inhibition induced by stimulation of pudendal nerve afferents. Neurourol Urodyn 5: 381–389

Vorstman B, Schlossberg S, Kass L, Devine CJ (1986) Spinal nerve root surgery for urinary bladder reinnervation. Neurourol Urodyn 5: 327–333

Vorstman B, Schlossberg S, Landy H, Kass L (1987) Nerve crossover techniques for bladder reinnervation: animal and cadaver studies. J Urol 137: 1043–1047

Wardrope J, Wilson DH (1986) Peripheral nerve grafting in the spinal cord: a histological and electrophysiological study. Paraplegia 24: 370–378

Webb DR, Fitzpatrick JM, O'Flynn JD (1984) A 15-year follow-up of 406 consecutive spinal cord injuries. Br J Urol 56: 614–617

Subject Index